# Dietary Triggers
# for
# Migraine

Agnes Peg Hartnell, EdD, RD

G. Scott Tyler, MD

Cover: Original sculpture by Peg Hartnell. Cover design by Jan Hancock.

**Publisher's Cataloging in Publication**
*(Prepared by Quality Books Inc.)*
Hartnell, Agnes Peg
  Dietary Triggers for Migraine / Agnes Peg Hartnell,
  G. Scott Tyler
       p.     cm.
  Includes index.
  ISBN 0-9649229-0-8
  1. Migraine—Nutritional aspects. 2. Diet in disease.
  I. Tyler, G. Scott. II. Title.
  RC392.H37 1996                    616.8'57'071
                                    QBI96-20012

$14.95

Printed in the United States of America

**Hancock Resources**
P.O. Box 33308
Phoenix, AZ 85067-3308, USA

# Acknowledgements

We are indebted to Millie Krull and AAA Copycraft for their skill and industry in deciphering the manuscript and rendering a coherent product. Much gratitude is also due to the dietitians who gave permission to use their original materials which we adapted for the cookbook; especially Pam McCarthy, RD, and Ann Moore Allen, RD.

Current and varied periodical references were provided by Frances Reay, Cathy Corak, Marie Shultz, Mary Rice, Karolyn Frye, Sue Zevan, and others.

Also, we owe much gratitude to Elaine F. Kvitka, RD, Jan Hancock, MA, Louise Beckwith, RN, and Joanne M. Hagmann, home economist, who cheerfully proofread, reviewed, and offered editing advice. Our thanks to Lee Fischer and Karin Wade of The Book Studio who helped to bring this project to fruition.

Thank you all very much!

# Dedication

For all their special help, and love—the Verlin P. Jenkins family, Hanna Hartnell, Jan, Brian, and Shannon Hancock

# Contents

## TABLES & CHARTS

# PART ONE

# Migraine Prevention

## Getting it Right,
## Getting it Done!

# Introduction

Do you have frequent, severe headaches, including migraine? Do you know anyone else who does? Ninety percent of Americans do.

Each year headache sufferers spend about $400 million on over-the-counter medications. Studies indicate that half of the 45 million Americans who suffer headaches do not seek a physician's help. Nearly 90 percent could be treated successfully. [1]

After treating headache patients for thirty years, Scott Tyler, M.D., became convinced that certain foods could trigger headaches. Within the last few years, as Chapter 1 shows, many other physicians are reaching the same conclusion.

Dr. Tyler and Dr. Agnes Peg Hartnell, a registered dietitian and home economist, have collaborated to compile this headache prevention book.

In this book none of the twelve, established headache-triggering foods is used in the recipes. Two additional food lists, that have been found dangerous to some, are marked with an asterisk(s) in the recipes for your safety.

This headache control book, as far as we can determine, is the first and only book written for today's life style with three types of recipes:

- Quick and Easy (take no longer to prepare than eat). This type may include microwave instructions.
- Prepare now - Reheat later
- Specialty (Gourmet/Creative) Recipes.

In this book we write of migraine and headaches without necessarily differentiating one from the other. There possibly is no difference in the cause of the migraine and other types of headaches such as cluster and muscle contraction or tension headaches anyway: *dietary management applies to them all!*

Your physician may not be familiar with the principles underlying the program, so you may wish to show this book to that physician so you may work together using these concepts.

For all migraine patients, daily exercise, eating breakfast, sufficient sleep and other healthy wellness habits may be as good as medicine in reducing the frequency and severity of migraine headaches (less bodily trauma).

For those migraine sufferers who become too incapacitated to cook, consider having on hand a stockpile of selected baby foods—nutritious, convenient, portable, easy-to-eat and free from salt and additives.

What about the recently approved migraine cure, sumatriptan and others awaiting government acceptance? [2] Most patients prefer prevention to cures, especially with new medications that have not stood the test of time and may have potentially harmful side-effects. Consult your doctor for diagnosis and treatment.

What about the theory that migraine "washes" from decreased blood flow (spreading electrical depression) from a small region at the rear of the brain? Further research is required, but it is interesting to note that in the animal model, one of the three stimuli was amino acids (protein particles) as found naturally in certain foods.[3]

Most readers will probably want to read the first chapter and then go directly to Chapter 4 for the foods to avoid, and the recipes that follow in Part II.

For those who wish further knowledge, Chapter 2 explains *how* food ingredients cause headaches. Chapter 3 adds information about medications and other non-food substances that can bring on headaches.

The following more than two hundred recipes are designed to fit into your total program for headache reduction. Choose one of the recipes to start with today - Bon Appetit!

## Chapter One

# IS DIET A POSSIBLE CAUSE OF HEADACHE?

Fortunately for you and all of us there has been an explosion in the amount of knowledge about the role of nutrition and health, including headaches, in the past decade!

As with any newer information, how can a person judge whether it's fact or fiction? You may be wondering why the relationship between headaches and diet is not now universally recognized.

One test of any health claim's (including headache's) fact or fiction is checking the scientific studies that back up the claim. [1] Therefore, it is important to know the reputations of the scientist(s) who conducted the study and whether the study is published in a reputable scientific journal. These journals do not publish a study unless it has been reviewed and passed by other researchers.

Medical breakthroughs are broadcast and published in both the scientific and popular media and press. The remainder of this chapter reports reputable studies from both types of publications. Their sources are also given so that you can read the original and check the connection between food and headaches.

According to *Taber's Medical Dictionary,* migraine is defined as an attack of headache usually accompanied by disordered vision and gastrointestinal upset . . . and may be the result of dilation of the cranial (brain) arteries . . . and may be precipitated by allergic hypersensitivity or emotional disturbances. [2]

This 1985 definition is more generous than many previous references that found no relationship between headaches and allergic hypersensitivity. [3, 7] Emotional or physical disturbances, causing stress, had been widely accepted as a cause of headache; most practitioners now accept also that heredity is an important factor.

However, "Headaches can be triggered by what you eat,"

according to John Brainard, M.D., in *Control of Migraine*. [4]

Another medical doctor, William J. Stump in 1984, contributed to a headache cookbook whose main emphasis was on diet and the role played by food in causing headaches. [5]

Neil Solomon, M.D. former *Los Angeles Times* health columnist, advised in 1990 that headaches might be helped by diagnosis and treatment involving food, chemical, mold, and yeast allergies for hypersensitivities. In one of his columns, Dr. Solomon pointed out the individuality of headache sufferers: men and women respond differently to the same drug (or food) so "it is possible a different medication or diet would be prescribed for each." Air flights are also related to headaches, as well as foods heavily salted with additives: "If you are subject to food-induced headache attacks, it would also be a good idea for you to bring along some food of your own on air travel trips. The in-flight food ordinarily contains a number of additives for flavor and these chemicals can precipitate a headache." [6]

In 1988, *Environmental Nutrition*, a professional newsletter of diet, nutrition, and health, carried an article headed *"Can Migraines Be Managed Through Diet? Foods That May Be To Blame."* While the exact causes of headaches remain unclear, a large number of experts believe that certain components of the diet may trigger headache episodes. "Food additives and some naturally-occurring substances in food could be the culprits . . ." Accompanying charts list foods headache sufferers should avoid, food additives, and eating patterns. [7]

Another medical practitioner, Lorain Stern, in a popular magazine *Women's Day,* wrote in their Medical Facts Guide that certain foods may contribute to migraines, most notably foods containing tyramines. [8]

Seymour Diamond, M.D., a specialist in headaches, has noted that in some persons low glucose blood levels can set off a headache attack. [9]

Registered dietitians, in addition to medical physicians, have written of diet and meal plans to control headaches. Betty Wedman, R.D., says that one rule of thumb for headache sufferers is: the more simple and natural the food, the less likely it will contain chemicals or salt that could cause an allergic (histamine) response. [10]

Carol A. Foster, M.D., of Valley Neurological Headache Clinic listed a change in diet as one of the effective tools for treatment of headaches at an exhibit on a two-year national tour that started at the National Museum of Health and Medicine in Washington, D.C. with a kick-off by former U.S. Surgeon General C. Everett Koop. [11]

And finally, some words from Joel Saper, M.D., director of the Michigan Head Pain and Neurological Institute in Ann Arbor and author of the 1987 Warner paperback *Help for Headaches:* What's really important is the change that's occurring in the scientific attitude about who gets headaches and why:

"Most headaches are due to disturbances in brain chemistry. That refines earlier views which blamed headaches on swelling of blood vessels or muscle tension. These changes can be involved, but they are triggered by quirks in the brain's messenger chemicals, according to the new view."

Dr. Saper points out that genetics make some people more susceptible than others. However, other factors such as medicine and food also play a role. He concludes that the new understanding of headaches is taking them out of the realm of psychological illness and putting them in the realm of a genetically determined (80%) biological illness.

In his advice on headaches, this question is included: Look at past headaches and keep notes on future ones and see if there's a pattern as to when they occur . . . after eating certain foods or taking certain medicines? Drinking something with caffeine or alcohol? . . . cigarettes? [12]

Thus, there have been many different approaches to headaches through history. And no doubt there will be new recommendations in the years and decades to come.

The recipes recommended in this book, high in natural foods and free of additives, can be of great benefit to headache sufferers and to all the members of their family.

Hopefully this review will encourage you to try a new lifestyle, one that is free from the dietary triggers of headaches.

# Chapter Two

# WHY SOME FOODS PRODUCE MIGRAINES

*(Skip this chapter unless you really want to know! Do show this book to your professional medical, dietetic or other health counsellor.)*

Some people, more often than not because of genetic inheritance, lack the ability or dietary enzymes to change some chemicals into harmless nutrients or chemicals in the body.

These chemicals can be found in certain medications or naturally, in some foods.

These particular drugs or foods, if not prevented by prior medications, can act as *messengers (headache triggers)*:

(1) irritating agents (like pollen can cause hay fever), or

(2) blood vessel constrictors/dilators *(pressor agents)* or blood pressure reactors.

The head's bony skull cannot expand to accommodate the swelling of the circulatory system. Either of these changes can trigger a headache.

The brain itself isn't hurting, because the brain has no nerves for experiencing pain. However, the arteries in the brain do have pain nerves; these pain signals can be transferred to the conscious center of the brain with every heart beat. [1]

What are the chemicals in foods or medications that can produce headaches in sensitive individuals? One way that specifically irritating foods was discovered was through the introduction of an anti-depressant medication (MAOI)* that hampered the action of an enzyme system in the liver that "digested" one of the brain's messenger chemicals, serotonin.

Normally, the liver changes the potentially harmful serotonin, found in some foods, into a harmless substance. "However, in the presence of this anti-depressant medication, MAOI, the body's defenses against serotonin are removed. If serotonin isn't neutralized by the body, its effect might be enhanced 100-fold. The

* monoamine oxidase inhibitor

patient develops a serious increase in blood pressure, headache, and even brain hemorrhage." [2]. The serotonin-sensitive individual can react the same, even without the MAOI inhibitor medication.

In addition to serotonin, other potent headache messengers include protein particles such as tyramine, tyrosine, dopamine, caffeine, glutamine, histamine, phenylethylamine, fermented foods, yeasts, and aged foods where protein breakdown occurs. The bacteria themselves, which are involved in the breakdown of protein, are capable of acting as headache trigger agents, too.

"The irritating content generally increases with the aging process of any protein-rich food and may undergo protein degradation given contamination and sufficient storage time. Cooking of degraded protein does not destroy the irritant. Recommend: perishable refrigerated items to be consumed within 48 hours of purchase." [3]

Thus in susceptible persons, diet-triggered headaches are linked to defective utilization of certain protein particles (amines). The resulting toxic products can also be caused by other foods which contain protein particles (without the action of bacteria), such as a few fruits and vegetables. Add sodium (commonly found in salt) and nitrates and nitrites (in smoked foods) for some people.

Some of the irritating foods contain weak triggering chemicals and in small quantities. These foods are unlikely to cause problems unless eaten in large amounts.

The offending chemical content can vary from product to product of the same class and even between samples of the same product. For example, the portions of cheese closer to the rind have a much higher tyramine content than those further from the rind. Dairy products, such as sour cream and yogurt, may or may not be irritating, depending upon their age and process of manufacture. [3]

The more simple and natural the food, the less likely it will contain chemicals that could cause an allergic response. Choose plainer dishes rather than dishes with sauces or casseroles when eating out.

To add to the confusion in discovering which particular foods a person is sensitive to, especially those whose families have a history of headaches, stress is a factor. Stress of any kind, especially emotional or physical, varies enough to lower the threshold for an attack one time and not for another with the same food. [4]

Many individuals find they can tolerate a small amount, approximately one-half cup (4 ounces) or less, of the offending food but not more, nor more often than once a week. However, there is no guarantee that the same foods will not produce a severe reaction in the future.

The opinions on the causes of headaches are not unanimous; but most headache specialists agree that diet and headaches have a strong connection. Frederick Freitag, M.D., says "a person who suffers four to five headaches a month can see a 50 percent reduction in attacks by simply controlling his or her diet." [5]

So what are the foods that contain the agents or chemicals that may have a connection? The lists could be divided into three categories:

(1) Foods Which Must Be Avoided by Most

(2) Foods To Be Consumed With Caution

(3) Foods Dangerous To Some Individuals.

### Foods Which Must Be Avoided by Most

Leading the list of avoidance is cheese (tyramine, bacteria, fermentation).

**Cheeses.** Limit *all* cheeses, including imitations which contain some natural cheese, except fresh cottage cheese, farmer's cheese, ricotta, and cream cheese. Avoid especially American, Blue, Brie, Boursault, Brick, Camembert, Cheddar, Emmentaler, Gruyere, Mozzarella, Provolone, Gouda, Swiss, Parmesan, and Roquefort.

**Beverages,** (aging, fermentation, tyramine, phenylethylamine, caffeine) beware of red wine, particularly Chianti, some beers and ales, liquors, cocoa, chocolate milk, excessive coffee, tea (over 2 cups each daily), and perhaps acidophilus milk and buttermilk.

**Chocolate** is double trouble because in addition to caffeine it contains the naturally occurring chemical agent phenylethylamine. However, all individuals do have different metabolic systems and many can tolerate cocoa, but not concentrated chocolate, as in sweets.

**Caffeine** is a weak pressor agent and in excessive amounts (over 2 cups of coffee or 4 twelve-ounce colas daily) may trigger a headache. Inversely, a headache may occur when excessive amounts of caffeine are suddenly stopped, as on a weekend. Theine, the stimulant in tea, affects a few.

**In wine,** red wine is usually made with grape pulp and seeds (phenolics) which are a source of protein and can serve as a contaminant to generate blood pressor messengers. White wine and vinegar are usually made without grape pulp or seeds and therefore may be tolerated.

The fermentation process in alcoholic beverages does not usually produce pressor agents, but any contamination can (and often does). The protein particle, tyramine, has occurred in Chianti and by-products of the fermentation process, called cogeners, which have been found in large amounts in Cognac and Scotch whiskeys.

**Red wine** is a particularly potent migraine headache producer because it also contains histamine, which causes blood vessel reactions. One sufferer rates brandy and liqueurs as the top two trouble makers, then wine, next bourbon or Scotch, and then gin. Vodka least of all because it is pure alcohol and water.

Some patients report headaches resulting from a rennet/milk powder pudding, yogurt or sour cream: consume with caution.

**Meats** (tyramine, bacteria, fermentation). All aged meats and fish that are smoked, salted, pickled or dried (such as herring, caviar), non-fresh meats (dry and semi-dry sausages, pepperoni, salami, aged corned beef, frankfurters, ham, bologna, and cold cuts) should be avoided.

Add to this list **liver** of all animals, especially chicken, liver paté, liverwurst, goose liver.

Include in the Must Be Avoided list any meats that are marinated, tenderized or aged over 24 hours; even some cooked meats or fish that have been refrigerated over 24 hours, such as canned tuna, sardines, or salmon.

**Meat extracts** are often concentrated from **aged** meats. They add flavor but also contain the offending chemicals. Check food labels on gravy mixes, commercial dinners, casseroles, soups, bouillon, canned stews, etc., for meat extracts.

Fresh meats, beef, lamb, poultry and fish are non-offenders although some find pork troublesome. Snails and artificial crab have been dangerous to some.

**Vegetables and Fruit Group** (dopamine) - Most items in this group are safe, but a few are on the definitely to-be-avoided lists. Fortunately these offending triggers are not too common favorites: soy beans, Italian green beans, lima beans, and broad bean pods, such as fava.

Some people also cannot freely eat legumes, such as peas, any beans, lentils, or Chinese pea pods. Definitely eliminate **sauerkraut** and other aged foods from the diet.

Other vegetables to be consumed with caution (1/2 cup, 4 ounces or less) are raw onions, beets (roots), and mushrooms.

**Fruits** (dopamines) - are not on the Must Be Avoided list! However, these may be a problem to some: avocado, ripe banana, citrus, red plums, canned figs, fresh pineapple, rhubarb, papaya, and raisins/dried fruit, dates. If you eat more than 1/2 cup (4 ounces) of any of these, it might be advantageous to try avoidance and determine the headache connection.

**Additives and Other Foods** (glutamine, nitrates). In addition to the food/beverage triggers, a common additive in over 2000 foods is monosodium glutamate. Glutamine is another chemical blood vessel messenger and to some people (approximately one out of four or six, depending upon the authority) nitrate and sodium (as in salt) also. Herbert Schaumberg, M.D. isolated monosodium glutamate as a cause of headache in his report, "The Chinese Restaurant Syndrome."

So many commercial products (to produce added flavor) contain the seasoning, monosodium glutamate, that home prepared foods may be preferable to commercially prepared mixes and eating out.

To many, salt-loaded foods can be a trigger. The most common offenders are not cooked foods where salt is mixed and diluted, but in highly salted items such as potato chips, nuts, crackers, pretzels, pickles, olives, anchovies, etc. Often these "appetizers" are taken on an empty stomach, plus a drink, plus a previous week of stress, which add up to a lost weekend with a headache.

If heavily salted foods are a headache trigger, then soy sauce, some salad dressings, Worcestershire sauce and other such seasonings fall into the salt load category. Flavorings such as curry powder and licorice are possibilities, too, for some.

Aspartame (phenylalanine) effects were shown in one study to cause a significant increase in headaches for sensitive individuals. This sugar substitute is being used more and more commercially and could add up to significant amounts in the diet. [6]

Nuts of all varieties may be a possible culprit to consider. Macadamia seem to be the least offending, with peanuts (and peanut butter) or coconut the most likely to trigger.

**Yeast.** The last offending agent on the Must Be Avoided list is the yeast group producing fermentation products. Therefore, avoid yeast extracts, yeast pills, and brewer's yeast. For some individuals freshly-baked yeasty breads that are still hot, including yeast-raised doughnuts, are dangerous.

By now you are probably wondering what you *can* eat! Thankfully, there is a longer list of allowed foods and foods in moderation which are included in the Food Purchasing Guide on page 27. The avoidance list may seem overwhelming; so concentrate on the allowed list of foods and the many appetizing recipes that can delight your taste buds.

# Chapter Three

## HOW SOME MEDICATIONS MAY PRODUCE HEADACHES

*(Another chapter for the health professional or the patient who really wants to know.)*

Significant amounts of a medication may enter the blood stream as early as five minutes after ingestion, according to John B. Brainard, M.D. As he says, "This rapid absorption into the body is logical, when one considers that nitroglycerine, an angina medication, is routinely given to patients as a tablet to be held under the tongue, where it is absorbed in a few minutes. This quick reaction accounts for the sudden onset of a headache (from certain medications), before the digestion of food which may take one-half to five hours." [1]

Medications that the individual is sensitive to should be identified, as well as foods, so that the headache (triggering) agents are blocked. These *agents* are many and varied, but in general may cause complex reactions in the blood or blood vessel constrictor/dilators in the head. [2]

Sometimes the reaction is caused by a dangerous combination of a food and a medication. [3, 4, 5, 6] Or, different medications will react with one another; therefore, it is important that the physician knows you and your case, as well as all your medications.

Betty Brackenridge, R.D., encourages the creation of a "super" supermarket shopping plan: consider not only the offending foods, but also the offending medication purchases. Before buying or taking a medication, ask your physician or pharmacist about the ingredients and check drug labels, both those at home as well as new ones. [9]

Another puzzle, entirely individual, concerns the enigma that one drug may be helpful to some, but precipitates headaches in another. [7, 8]

If **caffeine** is a headache trigger for you, then many stimulants and pain killers may be too. Inversely, some of these caffeine medications can be effective as headache preventatives to some individuals if taken daily. Other people find caffeine over-consumption or a related caffeine withdrawal can bring on a related headache. [1]

These findings indicate moderate use (2 cups daily) of caffeine; if you monitor the amount and frequency, the record may provide important information to you about the way your body reacts to this chemical (see page 20).

If **salt** (sodium) is a substance you're sensitive to, be aware that there exists a host of prescription and over-the-counter salt or sodium-containing products. [10]

### MEDICATIONS CONTAINING SODIUM [10]

- Analgesics
- Antacid-Analgesics
- Antacid Laxatives
- Antacids
- Laxatives
- Sleep-Aids
- Antacid Suspensions

Vitamin and mineral supplements may be additional sources of sodium also. Check the label!

### MEDICATIONS TO BE CHECKED FOR TRIGGERS

| | |
|---|---|
| Sleep Aids | Blood Pressure/Angina |
| Cold Medications | Stimulants |
| Nasal Decongestants | Vitamin/Mineral Preparations |
| Cough Suppressants | Antacids |
| Pain Pills | Laxatives |
| Oral Contraceptives | Fish Oil Pills (inconclusive) |

Reactive agents to look for include caffeine, salt load (sodium), propranolol, nitroglycerine, codeine, amphetamines, serotonin, MAOI inhibitors (monoamine oxidase), licorice.

Three plants, mistletoe, viscum, and American mistletoe, should not be used in drugs (or beverages or foods), since they contain the toxic pressor B-phenylethylamine and tyramine.

Licorice in quantity can cause sodium retention, potassium loss, diarrhea and elevated blood pressure. [6]

As yet the evidence on fish oil medications is inconclusive as to their effect on headaches. [11]

With so many potent headache-triggers in medications, keeping a diary of your intake of all kinds, including *whatever* you imbibe in any way, may offer a clue to the cause of that headache.

**Oral contraceptives** may contain chemicals that *decrease* the brain messenger, serotonin (and its metabolites), as well as vitamin B6. A decrease in B6 could cause depression. Depression is relieved with a supplement of 20 to 40 mg B6 daily on a physician's advice.

**Depression medications,** if specifically prescribed as monoamine oxidase inhibitors, *increase* serotonin (tyramine) effects so that food containing tyramines should *not* be added to the intake.

**Alcohol-sensitive individuals** should beware of flavorings with high percents of alcohol; also some medications, such as cough syrups, may be potent.

Prescriptions containing propranolol and nitroglycerine (high blood pressure and angina medications) affect blood vessels and blood pressure. Also check cold prescriptions, nasal decongestants, sinus aids, asthma inhalants, cough syrups (codeine) and weight reduction products (amphetamines).

# CAFFEINE CONTENT OF SELECTED FOODS & BEVERAGES [6]

| | Caffeine Content (mg/fl oz.) |
|---|---|
| Coffee, tea, cocoa | Range |

**Coffee—roasted, ground, instant**

| | |
|---|---|
| Percolated | 8-34 |
| Drip | 11-35 |
| Decaffeinated | 0.2-0.4 |
| Instant coffee, decaffeinated | 0.4-1.6 |
| Instant coffee, percolated & drip | 6-35 |

**Tea & Cocoa**

| | |
|---|---|
| Bagged tea | 6-9 |
| Leaf tea | 6-10 |
| Instant tea | 5-6 |
| Cocoa | 2-7 |

## Soft Drinks

**Regular**

| | |
|---|---|
| Cola or Pepper | 2.5-3.8 |
| Decaffeinated Cola | trace - 0.015 |
| Lemon-Lime (clear) | 0 |
| Orange | 0 |
| Other Citrus | 0-4.5 |
| Root Beer | 0 |
| Ginger Ale | 0 |
| Other Regular | 0-3.6 |
| Diet Cola or Pepper | 0.1-4.9 |
| Decaffeinated Diet Cola | trace-0.015 |
| Diet Lemon-Lime | 0 |
| Diet Root Beer | 0 |
| Other Diets | 0-3.6 |
| Club Soda, Seltzer, Sparkling Water, Tonic | 0 |

**Chocolate**

| | |
|---|---|
| Chocolate bar, 30 g. | 4 |
| Milk chocolate, 1 oz | 1-15 |
| Sweet chocolate | 5-35 |
| Chocolate milk, 8 oz | 2-5 |
| Baking chocolate, 1 oz | 8-118 |

Caffeine, theophylline, and theobromine are xanthine derivatives. Concurrent use may increase central nervous system stimulation and cause other additive toxic effects.

*Chapter Four*

# MANAGING MIGRAINE THROUGH DIET

## TWELVE FOODS TO BE AVOIDED BY MIGRAINE SUFFERERS

*These foods are **not** included in the recipes in this book.*

1. All cheeses including "imitation", except cottage cheese, farmer's cheese, ricotta, and cream cheese.

2. All *aged* meats and fish that are smoked, salted, pickled or dried (such as herring, caviar); non-fresh meats (dry or semi-dry) sausages, pepperoni, jerky, salami, frankfurters, hot dogs, aged corned beef.

3. Meats tenderized or marinated over 24 hours; even some refrigerated fresh or cooked meats within 24 hours.

4. Liver of all animals, liverwurst, liver patés.

5. Meat extracts such as gravy mixes, etc.

6. Lima, soy, fava, or broad bean pods, Italian bean pods, Chinese pea pods, lentils (check labels; ask when eating out).

7. Yeast extracts, brewer's yeast, freshly baked hot yeast products, like bread, rolls, doughnuts, etc.

8. Oriental soup stocks, bean paste (miso) and pickled foods (kimchee).

9. Chocolate, cocoa, cocoa butter.

10. Sauerkraut and other *aged* foods.

11. Red wines, Chianti, burgundy, sherry and vermouth.

12. Some hard liquor and liqueurs.

# FOODS DANGEROUS TO
# SOME INDIVIDUALS

*(Marked with a single asterisk in the recipes.)*

* Coffee, tea & other caffeine-containing beverages
* Fresh pineapple
* Curry powder
* Salad dressing  (check label for triggers)
* Rennet tablets
* Raisins & dried fruits, dates
* Imitation crab
* Coconut
* Canned figs
* Ham, bacon, pork
* Worcestershire sauce
* Licorice
* Mushrooms
* Snails
* Beet (roots)
* Salt load
* Rhubarb
* Hydrolyzed vegetable protein (check labels)
* Vanilla and other flavorings, especially if high percentage of alcohol.

Dried fruits, such as raisins, dates, etc., are not usually troublesome if fresh. Therefore, avoid the aged, hard, perhaps fermented product.

Some individuals report sensitivity to aspartame; milk and vitamin C preparations including multi-vitamin pills (if sensitive to citrus fruits).

Note: *Cooking does not usually eliminate triggering agents!*

# FOODS TO BE CONSUMED
# WITH CAUTION

*(Marked with a double asterisk in the recipes.)*

** Monosodium glutamate

** Soups made with instant soup powders

** Citrus fruit, particularly orange juice, perhaps lemon

** Soy sauce

** Ripe avocado

** Banana, particularly overripe

** Yogurt, sour cream, acidophilus milk and buttermilk

** Fresh raspberries

** Peanuts and some other nuts, except macadamia

** Distilled spirits, including white wine

** Red plums

** Onions, raw, cooked, dried

*The two trigger foods most often marked with asterisks in the recipes are onions and lemons,* because they are used the world over to enhance flavor. However, if used in amounts less than 1/2 cup they usually can be successfully tolerated by the headache-prone.

"The most definitive way of dealing with the diet is to eat nothing that is on the second or third list for the period of time in which you would expect to have three or more headaches. If it then appears to be successful, the dieter may re-enter certain favorite items such as *bananas* or *white wine,* one or two things at a time, in an attempt to liberalize the diet. Return of headache or the warning signs should be fair notice to discontinue suspect items immediately." [6]

# INTRODUCTION TO RECIPES

The rewards of using a headache cookbook are varied and many. To begin with there can be more freedom from headaches.

It's wonderful to be in control of triggering a headache rather than a headache's controlling what you do. And then there's comfort in knowing the agents you should avoid.

To top all this off, most recipes are quick to prepare. They have been tested and prepared by students in class laboratories, dietitians, or home economists.

While you and your cookbook are new to each other, allow three days between headaches before introducing a new ingredient (agent) for testing.

While most users of recipes value them for their freedom from headaches, it is likely that the absence of commercial additives, emulsifiers, preservatives, etc. makes the foods nutritionally superior to "fast" foods, purchased or prepared. Bearing in mind that food costs constantly escalate, recipes and menus are realistically geared to economy, too, whenever possible.

Tips and tables are included for nutritional substitutions and values of some common ingredients, shopping and meal plan guides, etc. Also note that heating times in microwave ovens may require adjustment since ovens vary.

Each recipe has its calorie, cholesterol, fat and sodium content listed. In recipes with egg substitutes and/or eggs, the nutritional analysis is based on the egg substitute. If you use whole eggs, see page 30 for conversion values.

Within each category, recipes are divided into the following preparation types.:
- Quick & Easy
- Prepare Ahead
- Specialty (Gourmet/Creative) Style

As you become more familiar with your recipes, and foods to avoid, you'll find yourself able to organize and prepare many meals of excellent variety and delectable taste for yourself and others. You'll be able to shop faster, and plan and prepare meals faster as you become familiar with the recipes and the foods you want to avoid because they trigger your headaches.

Now, here's how to begin: Read through the **Food Purchasing Guide** on page 27. This information is an excellent guide in helping you make your food purchases. Make a copy of it and take it with you when shopping. Avoid the offending foods listed, and buy foods that are in the "foods allowed" column.

To help you keep your headache control planning simple, **Meal Plans** are shown on the pages following the Food Purchasing Guide. Many of the recipes for the foods in the Meal Plans are included in the recipe section of this book.

You can mix or match as you desire, depending on which foods you especially enjoy.

The main factor to remember is keep a *record* of what you've eaten so you can quickly identify a food that triggered a headache. (That's always easier if you follow a meal plan.)

A full page chart like the one shown below, follows on the next page. Photo copy the full page chart and record your weekly intake.

**FOOD INTAKE PLAN AND RECORD**

WEEK OF: _____

| MONDAY | TUESDAY | WEDNESDAY | THURSDAY | FRIDAY | SATURDAY | SUNDAY |
|--------|---------|-----------|----------|--------|----------|--------|
|        |         |           |          |        |          |        |
|        |         |           |          |        |          |        |
|        |         |           |          |        |          |        |
|        |         |           |          |        |          |        |
|        |         |           |          |        |          |        |
|        |         |           |          |        |          |        |
|        |         |           |          |        |          |        |
|        |         |           |          |        |          |        |
|        |         |           |          |        |          |        |
|        |         |           |          |        |          |        |
|        |         |           |          |        |          |        |
|        |         |           |          |        |          |        |

| Headache(s) _____ | Headache(s) _____ | Headache(s) _____ | Headache(s) _____ | Headache(s) _____ | Headache(s) _____ | Headache(s) _____ |
| (Time(s) _____ | Time(s) _____ | Time(s) _____ | Time(s) _____ | Time(s) _____ | Time(s) _____ | Time(s) _____ |

Reproduction of this chart is permitted.

# FOOD INTAKE PLAN AND RECORD

WEEK OF: _____

| | MONDAY | TUESDAY | WEDNESDAY | THURSDAY | FRIDAY | SATURDAY | SUNDAY |
|---|---|---|---|---|---|---|---|
| | | | | | | | |
| | | | | | | | |
| | | | | | | | |
| | | | | | | | |
| | | | | | | | |
| | | | | | | | |
| | | | | | | | |
| | | | | | | | |
| | | | | | | | |
| | | | | | | | |
| | | | | | | | |
| | | | | | | | |
| | | | | | | | |
| | | | | | | | |

Headache(s) ____ Headache(s) ____ Headache(s) ____ Headache(s) ____ Headache(s) ____ Headache(s) ____ Headache(s) ____
(Time(s) ____ Time(s) ____ Time(s) ____ Time(s) ____ Time(s) ____ Time(s) ____ Time(s) ____

Reproduction of this chart is permitted.

# FOOD PURCHASING GUIDE

| Food Group | Foods Allowed | Foods in Question | Foods to Avoid |
|---|---|---|---|
| BREADS, CEREALS & GRAIN PRODUCTS | Most breads. Cooked and cold cereals, muffins, biscuits, pancakes, waffles, cookies and cake made without chocolate. | Hot yeast-raised breads. Ready-to-eat cereals or crackers with nuts, coconut, or dried fruits, high salt or sodium. Some commercial mixes. | Bakery and cereal products with chocolate. Questionable foods if sensitive. Crackers with cheese, MSG, yeast, extract flavorings. |
| FRUITS | Any others not listed. | Dried fruits. Ripe banana, avocado, red plums, fresh raspberries, papaya, rhubarb, pineapple. More than 1 citrus daily. | Any of the fruits in question in the canned state if the fresh fruit triggers a migraine. |
| VEGETABLES | Any others not listed. | Raw and cooked onions, beets (roots), eggplant, kimchee (pickled vegetable). | Broad bean pods, Italian bean pods, Chinese pea pods. Sauerkraut. |
| LEGUMES & NUTS | Unsalted, fresh macadamia nuts. | Peanuts and peanut butter. Other nuts. Beans and lentils. | |
| MEAT, POULTRY, FISH | Canned tuna in water, fresh beef, lamb, veal, poultry, fish. | Canned fish (heavily salted), pork, ham, bacon, snails, imitation crab. | All aged meats including salted, smoked, dried, pickled, marinated or tenderized; sausage, pepperoni, corned beef, liver and meat extracts, patés. |
| MILK & DAIRY PRODUCTS | Whole, low fat and skim milk, cottage cheese, ricotta and cream cheese. | Yogurt, sour cream, acidophilus milk, buttermilk (1/4 to 1/2 cup) depending upon age and manufacturing process. | Chocolate milk, aged cheeses of all kinds, natural or imitation. |
| FATS & OILS | Any others not listed. | Salad dressings and mayonnaises with wine vinegar, salt, or additives. | |
| ALCOHOLIC BEVERAGES | White wine, vodka (if tolerated or desired) | | Beer, ale, red wines, Chianti, sherry, vermouth, distilled hard liquor, liqueurs. |
| OTHERS | **Vinegar, eggs, hard candy, vanilla ice cream, non-cola soft drinks, tapioca. | MSG, soy sauce, Worcestershire sauce, curry powder, vanilla*, licorice, all caffeine-containing beverages, hydrolyzed vegetable protein, nitrites, nitrates, bouillon cubes, heavily salted foods, aspartame. | Chocolate and products containing chocolate. Marinades and tenderizers, yeast extracts and brewer's yeast. All aged foods. |

* imitation vanilla  —  ** white vinegar

Reproduction of this page is permitted.

# MEAL PLAN GUIDE

| BREAKFAST | LUNCH | DINNER | SNACKS |
|---|---|---|---|
| *Breakfast Burrito*<br>Kiwi | *Egg Salad Sandwich* | *Stir Fry Chicken & Broccoli*<br>(No MSG or Soy Sauce)<br>Rice | *Caramel Custard* |
| *Jam Toast Triangles* | *Chicken Pot Pie* | *Pasta Primavera with Salmon* | *Fudgy Brownies* |
| Oatmeal and Milk<br>1/2 Banana | *Savory Beef Burger* | *Texas Meat Loaf*<br>Baked Potato<br>Steamed Carrots | Pear |
| *French Toast*<br>Strawberries | *Taco Salad* | *Turkey "Sausage" Patties*<br>Mixed Salad Greens<br>*Italian Dressing* | *Poppy Seed Loaf* |
| Cottage Cheese on<br>English Muffin | *Chicken Vegetable Salad* | *Shrimp Sauté with*<br>*Dijon Mustard*<br>*Fruit Blintz* | *Health Nog* |
| *Omelet Primavera*<br>1/2 Grapefruit | Tuna Salad in Tomato<br>*Crunchy Bread Sticks* | *Favorite "Ham" Loaf*<br>*Harlequin Slaw*<br>*Pumpkin Bread* | *Lemon Love Notes* |
| Rice puffs and milk<br>Melon | *Turkey Chili*<br>*Whole Grain Muffins* | Beef Steak<br>*Wild Rice Casserole* | *Sweet Potato Chips* |

Items listed in bold and italic are recipes in this book.

# TYRAMINE RESTRICTED DIET (MAO)

## BREAKFAST

| | |
|---|---|
| Fruit Juice | Kiwi Fruit | Cranberry Apple Juice |
| Cereal | Cream of Wheat | Oatmeal |
| Meat/Meat Substitute | Soft Cooked Egg | Soft Cooked Egg with Salsa |
| Bread - margarine | Toast - butter or margarine | Tortilla - butter or margarine |
| Milk | Milk | Milk |
| Beverage | Coffee or Tea | Coffee or Tea |

## DINNER — NOON OR EVENING MEAL

| | |
|---|---|
| Meat/Meat Substitute | Broiled Beef Patty | Boiled Pinto Beans with Salsa |
| Potato/Potato Substitute | Mashed Potatoes | |
| Vegetable and/or Salad | Steamed Spinach | Steamed Spinach |
| Dessert | Gelatin Cubes | Flan (Caramel Custard) |
| Bread - margarine | Whole Wheat Bread with margarine | Flour Tortilla |
| Beverage | Coffee or Tea | Coffee or Tea |

## SUPPER — NOON OR EVENING MEAL

| | |
|---|---|
| Soup or Juice | Consommé | Broth |
| Meat/Meat Substitute | Roast Chicken | Roast Chicken |
| Vegetable and/or Salad | Peas | Peas |
| Bread-margarine | Creamy Coleslaw | Creamy Coleslaw |
| Dessert | Biscuit with margarine | Fresh Apple |
| Milk | Baked Apple | Flour Tortilla |
| Beverage | Milk | Milk |
| | Coffee or Tea | Coffee or Tea |

(See Nutritional Analysis on next page)

Adapted from Ann Moore Allen, Arizona Diet Manual.[7]

*Charts* — 29

# Nutrient Analysis of Tyramine Restricted Sample Menu

| | | | | | |
|---|---|---|---|---|---|
| Calories ...... 1700 cal | Vitamin A ..... 1371 RE | Calcium ........ 952 mg | Iron .......... 13 mg | Dietary Fiber . 16 gm | Folate ....... 337 mg |
| Protein ...... 102 gm | Vitamin C ..... 99 mg | Phos. ......... 1493 mg | Sodium ....... 2373 mg | Cholesterol ... 443 mg | Thiamin ..... 1.3 mg |
| Carb. ........ 176 gm | Niacin ........ 25 mg | Zinc ........... 12 mg | Pot. ......... 3040 mg | Fat ............ 68 gm | Riboflavin ... 1.9 mg |

# NUTRITIONAL CONVERSIONS OF FOUR RECIPE INGREDIENTS

## FAT

| | Calories | Salt | Cholesterol | Fat |
|---|---|---|---|---|
| Butter (1 Tbsp.) | 102 | 95 mg | mg | 11.5 g |
| Margarine (1 Tbsp) | 102 | 95 mg | | 11.5 g |
| Soft Stick (1 Tbsp.) | 80 | 79 mg | | 8g |
| Vegetable Oil (1 Tbsp.) | 120 | 70 mg | | 13.6 g |
| Cooking Spray (1 1/2 sec.) | 7 | 0 | 0 | 1 g |

## EGGS

| | Calories | Salt | Cholesterol | Fat |
|---|---|---|---|---|
| Egg Substitute (1/4 c.) | 25 | 80mg | 0 mg | 0 g |
| Egg (1 whole) | 70 | 60 mg | 240 mg | 5 g |

## MILK

| | Calories | Salt | Cholesterol | Fat |
|---|---|---|---|---|
| Whole (1 cup - 3/7%) | 157 | 119 mg | 35 mg | 8.9 g |
| 2% (1 cup) | 121 | 122 mg | 18 mg | 4.7 g |
| 1% (1 cup) | 102 | 123 mg | 10 mg | 2.6 g |
| Skim (1 cup) | 86 | 126 mg | 4 mg | .4 g |
| Buttermilk (1 cup) | 99 | 257 mg | 9 mg | 2.2 g |

## SALT

| | SALT (Sodium) | Potassium |
|---|---|---|
| Salt (1 tsp.) | 2300 mg | 0 |
| Garlic Salt (1 tsp.) | 2050 mg | Trace |
| Butter-Flavored (1 tsp.) | 1125 mg | 0 |
| Season All (1 tsp.) | 980 mg | 17 mg |
| Lite Salt (1 tsp. | 1100 mg | 1500 mg |
| No Salt (1 tsp.) | 1500 mg | 385 mg |

*PART TWO*

# Dietary Triggers for Migraine

# RECIPES

**Always check labels for dietary triggers!**

# APPETIZERS & BEVERAGES

# Chicken Paté

Prepare Ahead—Specialty

Makes 1 loaf—32 servings

** Onion

*Here's a paté, minus the liver, that you can indulge in to your heart's content.*

1-1/2 pounds boneless uncooked CHICKEN BREASTS, ground
1/2 cup finely chopped ONION**
6 Tbsp. EGG SUBSTITUTE or 2 EGGS
3 Tbsp. WHITE VINEGAR
1/2 tsp. BASIL LEAVES
1/8 tsp. ground BLACK PEPPER
1 cup finely chopped, peeled APPLE
1 cup dry BREAD CRUMBS
3 Tbsp. MARGARINE
1/2 tsp. THYME LEAVES
1/4 tsp. crushed fresh GARLIC

Thoroughly combine ground chicken, apple, bread crumbs, onion, eggs or egg substitute, 2 tablespoons margarine, vinegar, thyme, basil, garlic, and pepper. Grease a loaf pan with 2 teaspoons margarine (8 1/2 x 4 1/2 x 2 1/2). Press chicken mixture into pan. Dot with remaining margarine. Set loaf pan in shallow pan of water and bake at 350 degrees F. for one hour or until firm and pulling away from sides of pan. Drain excess liquid from pan. Cover and weight down paté while it is very hot. Cool slightly and then refrigerate, weighted, until well chilled.

MICROWAVE: Prepare chicken mixture as above, using a 5-cup microwave-proof ring mold. Cover. Microwave on HIGH (100% power) for 6 to 8 minutes, rotating 1/2 turn after 3 minutes. Weight and chill as above.

SERVING SIZE: 1/8" slice

CALORIES: 50    CHOL.: 12 mg   FAT: 1 g   SODIUM: 42 mg

* = Dangerous to Some    ** = Consume with Caution    (see Pages 22 & 23)

# Cucumber Canapés

**Makes 2 dozen**

*A bright and colorful, crunchy canapé that is
also cholesterol-lowering.*

**1/4 cup MARGARINE**softened
**24 (2-inch) BREAD ROUNDS**
**2 Tbsp.** *CREAMY MAYONNAISE*
  (see *SALADS*)
**6 CHERRY TOMATOES, thinly sliced**

**1 tsp. grated ONION ***
**24 slices CUCUMBER**
**3 Tbsp. chopped
  PARSLEY**

In small bowl, blend together margarine and onion. Spread rounds of bread with mixture. Top each with a cucumber slice and 1/4 tsp. *Creamy Mayonnaise.* Garnish with parsley and a tomato slice.

SERVING SIZE: 1 canapé

CALORIES: 41   CHOL.: 0    FAT: 2 g  SODIUM: 53 mg

# Sweet Potato Chips

**Makes 4 servings**

*This is delicious and flavorful and an excellent source of the
vegetable form of vitamin "A", beta carotene.*

**2 cups SWEET POTATOES, very thinly sliced**
**2 tsp. BUTTER**
**1 Tbsp. BROWN SUGAR**

Spread potato slices in microwave-safe dish. Sprinkle with water. Microwave on high 5 minutes. Mix butter and brown sugar and spread on slices. Microwave another 2 to 5 minutes. Let stand.

SERVING SIZE: 1/2 cup

CALORIES: 59   CHOL.: 5 mg   FAT: 2 gr  SODIUM: 21 mg

* = Dangerous to Some  ** = Consume with Caution  (see Pages 22 & 23)

# Individual Salmon Soufflés

Specialty

**Makes 16 appetizers**

**\*\* Scallions, lemon juice**

*Here's a healthy version for entertaining that's really different. This dish takes a bit of time, but it's well worth the effort.*

*SINGLE CRUST FLAKY PASTRY,* **doubled** (see *Desserts*)
1-1/4 cups **SKIM MILK**
1/4 cup **quick-cooking TAPIOCA**
1/4 cup **EGG SUBSTITUTE or 1 EGG**
1 Tbsp. **MARGARINE**
1/2 pound **RED SALMON, poached in water**
2 Tbsp. **minced PARSLEY**
2 Tbsp. **finely chopped SCALLIONS \*\***
1 Tbsp. **LEMON JUICE \*\***
1/2 tsp. **DRY MUSTARD**
4 **EGG WHITES, stiffly beaten**
1/8 tsp. **ground BLACK PEPPER**

Roll pastry into 16 (4-inch) circles. Mold on bottom side of muffin cups to make shells. Prick pastry and bake at 400 degrees F. for 10 minutes or until golden brown. Remove to wire racks to cool.

Combine skim milk, tapioca and egg substitute; let stand for 5 minutes. Bring to a boil; cook and stir until very thick, about 10 minutes. Remove from heat; stir in margarine.

Skin and bone poached salmon; flake meat. Combine salmon, scallions, parsley, lemon juice, mustard and pepper thoroughly and blend in cooked tapioca mixture. Stir 1/3 beaten egg whites into salmon mixture. Fold in remaining beaten egg whites. Spoon into pastry shells, mounding tops. Place on baking sheet; bake at 350 degrees F. for 30 to 35 minutes or until puffed and golden brown. Serve immediately.

SERVING SIZE: 1 appetizer

CALORIES: 190   CHOL.: 9 mg   FAT: 9 g   SODIUM: 105mg

\* = Dangerous to Some   \*\* = Consume with Caution   (see Pages 22 & 23)

# Spinach Balls

**Makes 36 spinach balls**

*This unusual recipe can be served as a terrifically tasty appetizer, or, as a great evening snack!*

**1 pkg. (10 oz.) frozen CHOPPED SPINACH, thawed and squeezed dry**
**1 Tbsp. MARGARINE, melted**
**3/4 cup EGG SUBSTITUTE, or 3 eggs**
**1 cup HERBED SEASONED STUFFING MIX**
**1 small ONION,** chopped

Preheat oven to 350 degrees F.   In medium bowl, combine spinach, stuffing mix and onion.  Blend in egg substitute and melted margarine.  Shape into 1-inch balls.  Place on lightly greased baking sheet. Bake at 350 deg.F. for 10 to 15 minutes. Serve hot.

MICROWAVE: Prepare as above.  Arrange 12 balls in 9-inch microwave-safe pie plate.  Microwave on HIGH (100% power) for 2-1/2 to 3 minutes. Rotate dish 1/2 turn after 1-1/2 minutes. Repeat with remaining spinach balls.

Tip:  Prepare ahead.  May be wrapped, frozen, then re-heated and served later.

SERVING SIZE: 1 spinach ball

CALORIES: 12     CHOL.: 0          FAT: 1 g   SODIUM: 33 mg

* = Dangerous to Some   ** = Consume with Caution   (see Pages 22 & 23)

# Stuffed Mushrooms

Specialty
*Mushrooms

Makes 1-1/2 dozen appetizers      **Onion, walnuts

*You might want to consider this appetizer as part of an hors d' oeuvre platter when company calls. The walnuts are not usually a trigger agent nor the small amount of onion.*

18 medium MUSHROOMS*, fresh
1/4 cup chopped ONIONS **minced
1/2 cup WALNUTS,** chopped
1/4 cup fresh BREAD CRUMBS
1/4 tsp. ground BLACK PEPPER
2 Tbsp. MARGARINE
1 clove GARLIC, minced
1 Tbsp. PARSLEY, chopped
dash ground RED PEPPER

Remove stems from mushrooms. Chop stems and set aside. Melt margarine in skillet. Mix in chopped mushroom stems, onion and garlic; saute until tender. Mix in walnuts, bread crumbs, parsley, black pepper and red pepper. Place mushroom caps on broiler rack. Stuff each cap with prepared filling. Bake at 350 degrees F. for 15 to 20 minutes or until done.

MICROWAVE: Remove stems from mushrooms; chop stems and set aside. In 1-1/2 quart microwave-proof casserole, microwave chopped stems, walnuts, margarine, onion and garlic on HIGH (100% power) for 2 to 2-1/2 minutes, stirring once. Stir in bread crumbs, parsley, black pepper and red pepper; stuff mushroom caps. Arrange stuffed mushrooms, 9 at a time, on a paper plate. Microwave on HIGH for 2 to 3 minutes, rotating 1/2 turn after 1-1/2 minutes. Repeat with remaining mushrooms.

SERVING SIZE: 1 stuffed mushroom

CALORIES: 43     CHOL.: 0     FAT: 3 g    SODIUM: 15 mg

* = Dangerous to Some    ** = Consume with Caution    (see Pages 22 & 23)

# Tortilla "Chips" & Low-Fat "Guacamole" Dip

Makes 2-1/2 cups  (40 Tbsp.)

Quick and Easy
** Lime juice

*Enjoy this low-fat dip without guilt!*

CORN TORTILLAS, cut into wedges
2 cups condensed GREEN SPLIT PEA SOUP, chilled
1 tsp. LIME JUICE**
1 small TOMATO, seeds removed
1/8 tsp. garlic powder or 1 fine minced GARLIC clove
1 can (4 oz.) chopped GREEN CHILES
1 Tbsp. chunky SALSA, (mild, med. or hot)
SALT or SALT SUBSTITUTE, if tolerated
TABASCO® to taste
GREEN FOOD COLORING

Cut corn tortillas into wedges, spray with non-stick product and bake in a 350 degree F. oven for 8 to 10 minutes or until crisp.  Sprinkle chips with light salt or salt substitute, if tolerated.

Combine the rest of the ingredients except Tabasco® and green food coloring in processor or blender.  Blend well until smooth and creamy.  Add a drop of coloring, one at a time, until nice and green.  Add Tabasco to taste.

Prepare ahead tip: Flavors enhance and dip holds well if prepared 2 to 6 hours ahead and refrigerated.

SERVING SIZE: 1 Tbsp.

CALORIES: 15    CHOL: 0 mg    FAT: .05 g    SODIUM: 62 mg

* = Dangerous to Some    ** = Consume with Caution    (see Pages 22 & 23)

# Nippy Dip

**Makes 1-3/4 cups**

**Prepare Ahead—Quick and Easy**
**\*\*Green onion, lemon juice, yogurt**

*High in calcium and can also be used as a sandwich spread!*

1 cup LOW-FAT COTTAGE CHEESE
3 Tbsp. finely chopped fresh PARSLEY
1/4 tsp. dried whole DILLWEED
3 Tbsp. reduced-calorie MAYONNAISE (check label)
SALT or SALT SUBSTITUTE to taste
3 Tbsp. minced GREEN ONIONS\*\*
1/2 tsp. LEMON JUICE\*\*
1/2 cup PLAIN NONFAT YOGURT\*\*

Combine cottage cheese and remaining ingredients in a bowl or blender; stir well. Cover and chill 3 hours. Serve with carrot and celery sticks or plain crackers.

Prepare ahead tip: Flavors enhance and dip holds well if prepared 2 - 6 hours ahead and refrigerated.

SERVING SIZE: 1 Tbsp.

CALORIES: 13     CHOL.: 1 mg     FAT: 0.5 gr     SODIUM: 48 mg

\* = Dangerous to Some     \*\* = Consume with Caution     (see Pages 22 & 23)

# Salsa Dip

**Makes 1-1/2 cups**

**Quick and Easy**
**\*\* Onion, lime juice**

*A southwestern dip to scoop up with tortilla or corn chips.*

**1 CUCUMBER, diced**
**3 TOMATILLOS (broil and remove skins)**
**1 Tbsp. WHITE VINEGAR**
**JUICE of 1 LIME \*\***
**1 tsp. JALAPEÑO PEPPER**
**1 TOMATO, chopped**
**1 Tbsp. chopped RED ONION\*\***
**pinch of SALT SUBSTITUTE, if tolerated**

Combine all ingredients in blender or food processor. Pulse until chunky.

SERVING SIZE: 1 Tbsp.

CALORIES: 6     CHOL.: 0     FAT: 1 g   SODIUM: 2 mg


# Red, White & Green Dip

**Makes 2 cups**

**Quick and Easy—Prepare Ahead**
**\*\* Onion, chives**

*Perfect for Christmas or any holiday.*

**12 oz. LOW-FAT COTTAGE CHEESE**
**1 Tbsp. RED PEPPER or PIMENTO, chopped**
**1/4 cup ONION,\*\* chopped**
**pinch of SALT and PEPPER**
**1 Tbsp. CHIVES,\*\* chopped**
**1 Tbsp. GREEN PEPPER, chopped**
**1/2 cup SKIM MILK**
**PAPRIKA**

Mix all ingredients except skim milk and paprika. Thin with the milk to desired consistency. Sprinkle with paprika.

SERVING SIZE: 1-1/2 Tbsp.

CALORIES: 14     CHOL.: 1     FAT: 0     SODIUM: 4 mg


* = Dangerous to Some   \*\* = Consume with Caution   (see Pages 22 & 23)

# Coffee Variations

Quick and Easy
*Coffee
**Orange rind

*If coffee is not a trigger for you, or decaf is safe, try these variations for a delicious drink.*

## Hot Spiced Coffee

**2/3 cup 2% low-fat MILK**
**1/4 tsp. GROUND ALLSPICE**
**3-1/2 cups hot brewed COFFEE***
**1 Tbsp. BROWN SUGAR**
**1 (4-inch) strip ORANGE RIND****
**1 (3-inch) STICK CINNAMON, crushed**

Combine milk, brown sugar, allspice, orange rind and cinnamon in a saucepan; bring to a boil. Remove from heat, and let stand 5 minutes. Line a colander with 4 layers of cheesecloth, allowing cheesecloth to extend over outside edges. Place colander over a large bowl or pitcher. Pour milk mixture into colander; discard spices. Add coffee to milk mixture; stir well. Serve immediately. Makes 4 cups.

## Spiced Iced Coffee

Pour 3 cups of hot, double-strength coffee over 2 cinnamon sticks, 4 cloves and 4 allspice berries. Let stand 1 hour; strain. Pour over ice in four tall glasses.

## Coffee Julep

Just add a dash of mint flavor to your iced coffee and serve in silver or aluminum tumblers, well frosted.

NOTE: Hot Spiced Coffee contains 33 calories per cup; 25 mg. sodium; and 3 mg. cholesterol.

* = Dangerous to Some   ** = Consume with Caution   (see Pages 22 & 23)

# Cranberry Cooler

Makes 1 serving

Quick and Easy
**Lemon juice

*A wonderfully refreshing drink that's beneficial as well!*

1/4 cup CRANAPPLE JUICE or use CRANBERRY or other
    CRANBERRY JUICE BLENDS
3/4 cup CLUB SODA
1/2 cup CRUSHED ICE
1 tsp. LEMON JUICE**

Combine cranapple juice, club soda and lemon juice. Stir and pour over crushed ice.

Tip: Team cooler with up to 3 cups "light" microwave popcorn. Check the package label for brands of popcorn that contain up to 2 grams or less of fat per 1 cup serving (to reduce calories).

SERVING SIZE: 1 cup

CALORIES: 42    CHOL.: 0    FAT: 1 g.    SODIUM: 1 mg.

# Creamy Mint Shake

Makes 2 servings

Quick and Easy
**Yogurt

*Such a refreshing, summer treat!*

1/2 cup CRUSHED ICE
1/4 cup SPARKLING MINERAL WATER
1/4 cup lightly packed fresh MINT LEAVES
1 (8 oz.) carton VANILLA LOW-FAT YOGURT** or milk-ice
    dessert
1 tsp. SUGAR
Fresh MINT LEAVES (optional)

Combine ice, mineral water, yogurt, sugar and mint leaves in container of an electric blender; cover and process 1 minute or until smooth. Serve immediately. Garnish with mint.

SERVING SIZE: 1 cup

CALORIES: 107    CHOL.: 6 mg.    FAT: 1.4 g.    SODIUM: 84 mg.

* = Dangerous to Some    ** = Consume with Caution    (see Pages 22 & 23)

# Health Nog

**Makes 8 servings**

*Almost a complete meal that tastes luscious and is luscious for your nutritional needs, too.*

**10 fresh or frozen STRAWBERRIES (if using frozen, let partially thaw)**
**1 8 oz. container EGG SUBSTITUTE**
**3 cups SKIM MILK**
**1/4 cup HONEY**
**1/3 cup frozen ORANGE JUICE CONCENTRATE****
**1 Tbsp. WHEAT GERM (optional)**

Place strawberries in bowl or blender/processor container. Mix or blend until smooth. Add skim milk, egg substitute, orange juice concentrate, honey and wheat germ (if desired). Mix or blend until well combined. Serve immediately.

SERVING SIZE: 3/4 cup

CALORIES: 106   CHOL.: 4      FAT: 1 g   SODIUM: 93 mg.

* = Dangerous to Some   ** = Consume with Caution   (see Pages 22 & 23)

# L'Orange Refresher

**Quick and Easy**
**Makes 1 serving**          **\*\*Orange juice, banana, yogurt**

*Use only 1/3 cup of ingredients that are dangerous for you.*

**1/2 cup ORANGE or PINEAPPLE JUICE\*\***
**1/4 cup 100% BRAN CEREAL®**
**1/2 medium ripe BANANA\*\***
**1/2 cup PLAIN NONFAT YOGURT\*\***
**1/4 cup SKIM MILK**

Place all ingredients in bowl or blender/processor container. Mix or blend until smooth. If using mixer, let bran soak in liquids for a few minutes first. Serve immediately.

NOTE: This drink <u>does</u> have 3 possible headache triggers for some individuals. Lowering the 1/2 cup measure to 1/3 cup may prevent a reaction, or simply delete if the item is aged.

SERVING SIZE: 1-1/4 cups

CALORIES: 264   CHOL.: 9 mg.   FAT: 3 g.   SODIUM: 282 mg.


# Skim Milk Hot "Cocoa"

**Quick and Easy**
**Makes 2 servings**          **\*Vanilla**

*With carob powder it almost tastes like chocolate!*

**2 Tbsp. CAROB POWDER**
**3 Tbsp. SUGAR or ARTIFICIAL SWEETENER**
**1-1/2 cups SKIM MILK**
**1/4 cup HOT WATER**
**1/8 tsp. VANILLA EXTRACT\***

In small saucepan blend carob powder and sugar; gradually add hot water. Cook over medium heat, stirring constantly, until mixture boils; boil and stir for 2 minutes. Add milk; heat thoroughly. Stir occasionally; do not boil. Remove from heat; add vanilla. Serve hot.

SERVING SIZE: 7 ounces

CALORIES: 161   CHOL.: 3 mg.   FAT: 1 g.   SODIUM: 97 mg.

* = Dangerous to Some   ** = Consume with Caution   (see Pages 22 & 23)

# Soups

# Salads

# Salad Dressings

# Double Potato Soup

**Makes 12 servings**

*This different version of potato soup can be made a main course by adding diced chicken breast and served with crusty French bread and fruit. This recipe will give you enough to freeze for another meal.*

1 Tbsp. MARGARINE
2 cans (14.5 oz. each) CHICKEN BROTH
4 large WHITE BAKING POTATOES, diced
1/8 tsp. GROUND BLACK PEPPER
1 medium YELLOW ONION\*\*,chopped
4 cups WATER
1 Tbsp. DILL WEED
1 large SWEET POTATO, peeled and diced

Melt margarine in a large soup pot. Add onion; cook over medium-low heat for 10 minutes. Add broth, water, potatoes and sweet potato. Bring to boil; reduce heat to medium-low and cook for about 20 minutes, or until potatoes are tender.

Remove soup from heat. When cool, puree liquids and solids in a blender or food processor (do in 3 batches). Return puree to pot. If consistency is too thick, add water until soup reaches desired consistency. Add pepper and dill. Keep warm over low heat.

SERVING SIZE: 1 cup

CALORIES: 73   CHOL.: 5 mg.   FAT: 5 g.   SODIUM: 1,000 mg.

\* = Dangerous to Some   \*\* = Consume with Caution   (see Pages 22 & 23)

# Egg Drop Soup

**Makes 6 servings**

Quick and Easy
**Scallions

1/4 tsp. TARRAGON LEAVES
4 packets or cubes low-sodium CHICKEN BOUILLON
2 SCALLIONS**,finely chopped
4 cups WATER
3 Tbsp. CORNSTARCH
3 Tbsp. EGG SUBSTITUTE, or 1 whole EGG, beaten

In medium saucepan, bring 3-1/2 cups water to a boil. Stir in chicken bouillon until dissolved. Combine cornstarch and remaining 1/2 cup water; add to bouillon, stirring constantly. Mix in tarragon. Cook and stir until thickened and boiling. Cook 1 minute longer. Reduce heat to low; gradually add beaten egg or egg substitute in a thin stream, without stirring. Cook for 30 seconds. Stir once or twice. Serve in bowls garnished with scallions.

SERVING SIZE: 3/4 cup

CALORIES: 28     CHOL.: 0     FAT: 0     SODIUM: 17 mg.


# Cabbage Soup

**Makes 6 servings**

Quick and Easy
**Onion

6 cups CABBAGE, chopped (or use market cole slaw)
1/4 tsp. CARAWAY SEED
1/8 tsp. PEPPER
1-1/2 tsp. SALT (optional)
1/4 tsp. DILL WEED
1 medium ONION**,peeled, sliced and separated into rings
4 cups hot WATER

Combine all ingredients; cover, simmer 15 to 20 minutes until cabbage and onion are tender.

SERVING SIZE: 1 cup

CALORIES: 59     CHOL: 0     FAT: 0     SODIUM: 142 mg

* = Dangerous to Some   ** = Consume with Caution   (see Pages 22 & 23)

# Creamy Romano Tomato Soup

**Makes 4 servings**                    **Quick and Easy**

*Remember when your mother brought you this comforting, tasty soup? Now yours is home-made and even better!*

**1-3/4 cups whole peeled TOMATOES, (14-1/2 oz. can) undrained**
**2/3 cup (6 oz. can) TOMATO PASTE**
**1 cup LOW-FAT MILK**
**1/2 cup low-salt canned CHICKEN BROTH (or use 1 BOUILLON CUBE)**
**fresh BASIL SPRIGS**

In blender or food processor, process tomatoes and juice, and tomato paste until blended. Stir in milk and chicken broth. Pour through sieve into medium saucepan to remove tomato seeds. Heat to serving temperature. Garnish with fresh basil.

SERVING SIZE: 1 cup

CALORIES: 106   CHOL.: 5 mg.   FAT: 1 g.   SODIUM: 350 mg.

# Lemon Soup

                         **Quick and Easy**
                           **\*\*Lemon juice**
**Makes 6 servings**
**1-1/2 cups WATER**
**2 cans (14.5 oz. each) CHICKEN BROTH**
**1 cup EGG SUBSTITUTE, or 4 EGGS, beaten**
**1/4 cup LEMON JUICE\*\***
**1/8 tsp. BLACK PEPPER**
**2 cups cooked WHITE RICE**
**1 pkg. (10 oz.) FROZEN SPINACH, thawed and drained**

Pour broth into pot and bring to a boil. Add rice, simmer 2 minutes. Combine egg substitute and lemon juice in a small bowl and mix well. Remove soup from heat.

Mix 2 cups of hot broth into egg mixture, stirring constantly. Pour mixture back into broth; stir in spinach. Add pepper; simmer for 5 minutes.

SERVING SIZE: 1 cup

CALORIES: 126   CHOL.: 2 mg.   FAT: 1 g.   SODIUM: 364 mg.

---

* = Dangerous to Some   \*\* = Consume with Caution   (see Pages 22 & 23)

# Mac & Beef Soup

*This soup is really a complete meal, yet easy to make, and even better the second time around, but not over 24 hours!*

VEGETABLE COOKING SPRAY
1/2 lb. lean GROUND BEEF
1/2 cup chopped GREEN PEPPER
1/2 cup chopped ONION**
1/2 tsp. dried OREGANO LEAVES, crushed
1/2 tsp. dried BASIL LEAVES, crushed
3 cans (10-3/4 oz. each) TOMATO SOUP
3 soup cans WATER
2 cups ELBOW MACARONI cooked in unsalted water
    and drained
2 tsp. LEMON JUICE**

Spray 6-quart pan with vegetable cooking spray. Over medium heat, cook beef, green pepper and onion with oregano and basil until beef is browned and vegetables are tender, stirring to separate meat. Spoon off fat.

Stir in soup, water, macaroni and lemon juice. Heat to boiling. Reduce heat to low. Simmer 20 minutes, stirring occasionally.

SERVING SIZE: 1-1/3 cups

CALORIES: 180   CHOL.: 21 mg. FAT: 3 g.  SODIUM: 367 mg.

* = Dangerous to Some   ** = Consume with Caution   (see Pages 22 & 23)

# Gazpacho

**Specialty**
**\*\*Onion, lemon juice**

*For hot summer days this southwestern soup is a natural; the green peppers, tomatoes, and tomato juice contribute valuable vitamin "C" for summer stress.*

3/4 cup TOMATO JUICE
2 Tbsp. LEMON JUICE\*\*
3 Tbsp. *SPICY TOMATO DRESSING* (see *Salads*)
2 Tbsp. finely chopped CELERY
1/4 tsp. GARLIC POWDER
1 Tbsp. chopped PARSLEY
3 cups fat-free BEEF BROTH or BOUILLON CUBES
1/3 cup finely chopped ONIONS\*\*
1/3 cup finely chopped GREEN PEPPERS
1 cup diced, peeled and cored fresh TOMATOES
1 tsp. SALT or SALT SUBSTITUTE
1/4 to 1/2 cup thinly sliced or diced CUCUMBERS

Combine all ingredients, except cucumbers, in a large bowl. Mix gently and refrigerate at least 4 hours. Garnish with cucumbers before serving.

SERVING SIZE: 3/4 cup

CALORIES: 35    CHOL.: 0    FAT: 1 g.    SODIUM: 944 mg.

\* = Dangerous to Some    \*\* = Consume with Caution    (see Pages 22 & 23)

# Turkey Minestrone

**Makes 8 servings**

*An old-fashioned, satisfying soup for a meal in itself. If any is left over, fill plastic drinking glasses, cover and freeze for individual servings with sandwiches another time.*

1 pkg. (about 1-1/4 lb.) fresh lean GROUND TURKEY
1 cup sliced CARROTS
1-1/2 tsp. dried BASIL LEAVES
1/4 tsp. PEPPER
3 (14-1/2 oz.) cans reduced-sodium or regular BEEF BROTH
1 pkg. (9 oz.) frozen cut GREEN BEANS
NON-STICK COOKING SPRAY
2 cups shredded CABBAGE
1/2 cup chopped ONION**
1/4 tsp. GARLIC POWDER
1 can (16 oz.) whole TOMATOES, undrained, cut-up
1 medium ZUCCHINI, diced
chopped fresh PARSLEY, if desired

Spray bottom of 6-quart saucepan or Dutch oven with non-stick cooking spray until well coated. Heat saucepan over medium-high heat about 30 seconds. Crumble ground turkey into pan. Cook and stir 3 to 5 minutes or until lightly browned. Add cabbage, carrots, onion, basil, garlic powder, pepper, beef broth and tomatoes; bring to a boil. Reduce heat to medium; cook 10 minutes, stirring occasionally. Add zucchini and green beans; cook an additional 8 to 12 minutes or until vegetables are tender, stirring occasionally. Sprinkle with chopped fresh parsley, if desired.

SERVING SIZE: 1-1/2 cups

CALORIES: 160   CHOL.: 48 mg.   FAT: 6 g.   SODIUM: 145 mg.

* = Dangerous to Some   ** = Consume with Caution   (see Pages 22 & 23)

# Simple Hot & Sour Soup

Quick and Easy
*Mushrooms

Makes 4 servings

**Onions, lemon juice

*You may have seen this favorite on Chinese menus; try it in your own kitchen for a change.*

2-1/2 cans (14.5 oz. each) CHICKEN BROTH
1 Tbsp. LEMON JUICE**
1 Tbsp. WHITE VINEGAR
1/2 cup LOW-FAT COTTAGE CHEESE
3 dried MUSHROOMS*, soaked in cold water for
    10 minutes and chopped
1/4 cup EGG SUBSTITUTE, or 1 EGG beaten
1 tsp. SESAME OIL
1/2 medium ONION**, finely chopped
1 Tbsp. TABASCO SAUCE
1 6 oz. can WATER CHESTNUTS
2 Tbsp. CORNSTARCH
2 Tbsp. cold WATER
1 GREEN ONION**, finely chopped

Heat oil in a saucepan. Add onions and cook until soft. Gradually add broth. Stir in lemon juice, tabasco sauce, vinegar, chestnuts, cottage cheese and mushrooms. Simmer for 15 minutes. Bring to boil. Mix cornstarch and water, add to boiling soup; stir until thickened. Add egg substitute, stir 1 minute. Simmer 2 minutes.

Ladle 1 cup of soup into a bowl, top with chopped green onions. Serve immediately.

SERVING SIZE: 1 cup

CALORIES: 148   CHOL.: 0   FAT: 5 g.   SODIUM: 374 mg.

* = Dangerous to Some   ** = Consume with Caution   (see Pages 22 & 23)

# Seafood Chowder

*This kind of dish was the origin of bouillabaisse. Thickened with pureed vegetables, instead of cream, serve this treat to yourself or the family. Freeze leftovers.*

1 lb. FLOUNDER or HALIBUT, cut in 2-inch pieces
1 cup chopped ONIONS\*\*, or sliced LEEKS
1 cup chopped CARROTS
3 cups peeled, diced POTATOES
1 BAY LEAF
1/2 tsp. SALT
1 can (10 oz.) chopped CLAMS, drained, liquid reserved
1 Tbsp. MARGARINE
2 cups LOW-FAT MILK
1 cup chopped CELERY
1/2 tsp. HOT PEPPER SAUCE
1/2 tsp. dried THYME

In 3-quart saucepot heat margarine over medium heat. Add onions, carrots and celery; saute 3 minutes. Stir in potatoes, bay leaf, salt and thyme. Combine reserved liquid from clams and enough water to equal 3/4 cup; add to saucepot. Simmer 15 minutes or until vegetables are tender. Puree half the chowder mixture and return to saucepot. Add fish; simmer 5 to 8 minutes or just until cooked. Stir in milk and clams. Heat through. (Do not boil.) Stir in hot pepper sauce.

SERVING SIZE: 1 cup

CALORIES: 160    CHOL.: 35 mg.   FAT: 3 g.   SODIUM: 390 mg.

---

\* = Dangerous to Some    \*\* = Consume with Caution    (see Pages 22 & 23)

# Zucchini Soup with Curry

**Makes 4 servings**

Easy
*Curry powder
**Onion, yogurt

2 Tbsp. OIL
4 medium ZUCCHINI, cut in
   1 inch cubes
1/2 cup sliced GREEN ONIONS**
1-1/2 tsp. CURRY POWDER*
1/8 tsp. PEPPER

1 can (13 oz.) CHICKEN
   BROTH
1 Tbsp. CORNSTARCH
1/2 cup APPLE JUICE
1 cup PLAIN NONFAT
   YOGURT**

In large saucepan heat oil over medium heat. Add zucchini, green onions and curry powder; sauté 5 minutes or until onions are tender. Add broth; reduce heat. Cover and simmer 30 minutes or until zucchini is tender. In small bowl mix cornstarch and apple juice until smooth; whisk into soup. Over medium heat, bring soup to a boil and boil 1 minute. Pour into blender or food processor; add yogurt and pepper. Blend or process until smooth. Serve hot or chilled. If reheated *do not boil!*

SERVING SIZE: 1 cup

CALORIES: 170   CHOL.: 5 mg.   FAT: 9 g.   SODIUM: 580 mg.

# Zucchini Soup

**Makes 2 servings**

Quick and Easy
**Onion

1-1/2 cups ZUCCHINI, sliced, plus 3 paper-thin slices
3 leaves of fresh BASIL, chopped, or 1/2 tsp. dried basil
1/2 cup chopped ONION**
1/2 cup CELERY
1/2 cup low-sodium CHICKEN BROTH
SALT and PEPPER to taste

Put all ingredients in one pot and simmer for 30 minutes. Put in blender and blend. Serve hot with slices of raw zucchini on top for garnish.

SERVING SIZE: 1 cup

CALORIES: 40   CHOL.: 0   FAT: 0   SODIUM: 253 mg.

* = Dangerous to Some   ** = Consume with Caution   (see Pages 22 & 23)

# Broccoli Pasta Salad

**Quick and Easy——Prepare Ahead**
**\*Mayonnaise**
Makes 4 servings (1/2 cup)   **\*\*Onion, lemon peel & juice**

3/4 cup REDUCED CALORIE MAYONNAISE* (check label)
1/2 cup cooked sliced CARROTS
1-1/2 cups (4 oz.) PASTA RUFFLES, cooked and drained
1 tsp. grated LEMON PEEL**
1/4 cup SKIM MILK
1/4 cup sliced GREEN ONIONS**
2 Tbsp. chopped PARSLEY
2 tsp. LEMON JUICE**
1 cup cooked (approx. 3 minutes) BROCCOLI FLORETS

In large bowl stir mayonnaise, onion, skim milk, parsley, lemon juice and lemon peel until smooth.  Add pasta ruffles, broccoli and carrots; toss to coat well.  Cover, chill.

*Prepare ahead tip:* Refrigerate 2 to 6 hours before serving.

SERVING SIZE: 1 cup
CALORIES: 140   CHOL.: 0   FAT: 5 g.   SODIUM: 130 mg.

# Crunchy 3-Bean Salad

**Quick and Easy**
Makes 6 servings   **\*Beans, if tolerated**

1 can (8-3/4 oz.) KIDNEY BEANS*
1 can (8-3/4 oz.) FRENCH STYLE GREEN BEANS*, drained
1 can (8-3/4 oz.) GARBANZO BEANS*
3/4 cup WHITE VINEGAR, mild
2 Tbsp. OLIVE OIL
1 tsp. GROUND OREGANO
1 Tbsp. SODIUM-FREE SALT
10 PEPPERONCINI PEPPERS, sliced
1 jar (20 oz.) PIMENTO

Combine beans, peppers and pimento in mixing bowl.  Mix together remaining ingredients in separate bowl.  Pour dressing over bean mixture.  Marinate 1 hour in refrigerator.

SERVING SIZE: 1 cup
CALORIES: 215   CHOL.: 0   FAT: 6 g.   SODIUM: 154 mg.

* = Dangerous to Some   ** = Consume with Caution   (see Pages 22 & 23)

# Chunky Tomato-Mushroom Salad

Quick and Easy
*Mushrooms
**Walnuts

Makes 6 servings

2 cups unpeeled TOMATO
  chunks (about 3/4 lb.)
1 Tbsp. chopped WALNUTS**
1 Tbsp. chopped fresh BASIL
2 tsp. VEGETABLE OIL

1 cup sliced fresh
  MUSHROOMS*
1 Tbsp. WATER
1 Tbsp. WHITE VINEGAR
1/8 tsp. SALT

Combine tomato chunks, mushrooms and walnuts in a bowl; toss gently. Combine basil, water, vinegar, salt and vegetable oil in a jar; cover tightly and shake vigorously. Pour over tomato mixture, toss gently.

SERVING SIZE: 1/2 cup

CALORIES: 37   CHOL.: 0   FAT: 2.4 g.   SODIUM: 54 mg.

# Chicken-Vegetable Salad

Quick and Easy
*Mayonnaise
**Onion

Makes 6 servings

2 cups chopped CHICKEN BREAST
1/2 cup diced CELERY
1/4 cup chopped PIMENTO
1/4 cup MAYONNAISE* (check label)
2 Tbsp. sliced SCALLIONS**
1/2 CUCUMBER, peeled and diced
1/4 cup diced GREEN PEPPER
1/2 cup WATER CHESTNUTS, drained and sliced
2 Tbsp. CAPERS
PAPRIKA

Toss chicken, cucumber, celery, green pepper, pimento, water chestnuts and scallions with mayonnaise. Serve on crisp salad greens, garnished with capers and paprika.

SERVING SIZE: 3/4 cup

CALORIES: 153   CHOL.: 40.5 mg.   FAT: 8.8 g.   SODIUM: 97.7 mg.

* = Dangerous to Some   ** = Consume with Caution   (see Pages 22 & 23)

# Couscous & Vegetable Salad

**Makes 8 servings**

*High in vitamin C, this winner can easily be prepared in advance to marry the flavors.*

1/4 cup VEGETABLE OIL
1/4 tsp. PEPPER
3 Tbsp. chopped FRESH BASIL or 3 Tbsp. chopped
    PARSLEY plus 1 tsp. dried BASIL
1 small RED or GREEN PEPPER, cut in matchstick strips
2 medium TOMATOES, diced
1 cup uncooked COUSCOUS
1 small ZUCCHINI, cut in matchstick strips
1 tsp. SALT
2 Tbsp. WHITE VINEGAR
1 small CLOVE GARLIC, minced or pressed
4 GREEN ONIONS\*\*,thinly sliced
2 Tbsp. sliced pitted ripe OLIVES

Prepare couscous according to package directions; cool. In large bowl combine oil, vinegar, basil, garlic, salt and pepper. Add couscous, tomatoes, zucchini, red pepper, green onions and olives; toss to coat well. Cover, chill.

SERVING SIZE: 1 cup

CALORIES: 90    CHOL.: 0    FAT: 8 g.    SODIUM: 370 mg.

---

\* = Dangerous to Some   \*\* = Consume with Caution   (see Pages 22 & 23)

# Cuke Salad

Prepare Ahead
*Mayonnaise
**Onion, walnuts

**Makes 8 servings**

1/2 cup chopped WALNUTS**
1/2 cup chopped CELERY
1 pkg. LIME SUGAR-FREE GELATIN
1/2 cup boiling WATER
1/2 cup LOW-FAT MAYONNAISE* (check label)
1 small ONION**, chopped
1 medium CUCUMBER, unpeeled and diced
1 Tbsp. WHITE VINEGAR
1 lb. LOW-FAT COTTAGE CHEESE
1 small can unsweetened PINEAPPLE BITS, including juice

Dissolve gelatin in hot water, add vinegar and remaining ingredients. Set in refrigerator until firm.

SERVING SIZE: 3/4 cup

CALORIES: 180   CHOL.: 3 mg.   FAT: 11 g.   SODIUM: 232 mg.

# Harlequin Slaw

Quick and Easy—Prepare Ahead
*Salad dressing
**Onion, lemon juice

**Makes 8 servings**

*This dish is just right for a picnic, no matter what the season.*

3 cups coarsely shredded RED CABBAGE
1/2 cup drained, canned, NO-SALT ADDED
    WHOLE KERNEL CORN
2 Tbsp. minced fresh PARSLEY
2 tsp. LEMON JUICE**
2 Tbsp. chopped GREEN ONIONS**
1/4 cup diced GREEN BELL PEPPER
3 Tbsp. LOW CALORIE SALAD DRESSING* (check label)

Combine all ingredients in a bowl; toss well.

SERVING SIZE: 1/2 cup

CALORIES: 36    CHOL.: 4 mg.   FAT: 1.3 g.   SODIUM: 15 mg.

* = Dangerous to Some   ** = Consume with Caution   (see Pages 22 & 23)

# Garden Fresh Tuna Salad

**Makes 8 servings**

*A colorful, flavorable combination of vegetables to add to an ordinary tuna salad dish. Minced garlic is available in small glass jars for convenience; find it in the produce department, and keep in the frig.*

2/3 cup REDUCED CALORIE MAYONNAISE* (check label)
2 Tbsp. SKIM MILK
1 lb. small NEW POTATOES, halved, cooked and cooled
1 YELLOW, RED or GREEN PEPPER cut in strips
1-1/2 cups halved CHERRY TOMATOES
1/4 cup minced RED ONION**
2 Tbsp. DIJON MUSTARD
1 CLOVE GARLIC, minced
2 cans (6-1/2 oz. each) WATER-PACKED TUNA, drained
1-1/2 cups fresh GREEN BEANS, cut and cooked  or, 1 pkg.
    frozen CUT GREEN BEANS, thawed)
LETTUCE

In large bowl combine mayonnaise, mustard, milk and garlic. Add potatoes, tuna, pepper, green beans, tomatoes and onion; toss to coat. Cover; chill. Serve on a bed of lettuce.

SERVING SIZE; 1 cup

CALORIES: 210   CHOL.: 10 mg. FAT: 7 g.   SODIUM: 340 mg.

* = Dangerous to Some   ** = Consume with Caution   (see Pages 22 & 23)

# Garden Pasta Salad

**Makes 6 servings**

*The yellow squash, cherry tomatoes and green peppers help
dress up this carbo-rich salad without unwanted calories.*

**3/4 cup REDUCED CALORIE MAYONNAISE\* (check label)**
**1/2 cup fresh PARSLEY LEAVES**
**1-1/2 cups (4 oz.) TWIST MACARONI, cooked and drained**
**1-1/2 cups CHERRY TOMATOES, quartered**
**2 Tbsp. WHITE VINEGAR**
**1 tsp. DRIED BASIL**
**1 CLOVE GARLIC**
**2 cups sliced YELLOW SQUASH**
**1 cup diced GREEN PEPPER**
**LETTUCE LEAVES**

In blender or food processor combine mayonnaise, parsley,
vinegar, basil and garlic; blend or process until smooth. In large
bowl combine macaroni, squash, tomatoes and green pepper.
Add dressing; toss to coat well. Arrange on lettuce-lined
platter.

SERVING SIZE: 1 cup

CALORIES: 190   CHOL.: 0      FAT: 6 g.  SODIUM: 160 mg.

\* = Dangerous to Some   \*\* = Consume with Caution   (see Pages 22 & 23)

# Green Grape & Apple Waldorf Salad

**Quick and Easy**
**\*Mayonnaise**
**\*\*Pecans, yogurt**

**Makes 4 servings**

*An old-time favorite variation (first made by the chef at the Waldorf-Astoria Hotel in the 1890s) that has been revived for the 1990s. Serve with meatloaf and brussel sprouts. Preparation time: 13 minutes.*

1 cup chopped unpeeled red APPLE
1/4 cup chopped CELERY
1 Tbsp. unsweetened APPLE JUICE
1 Tbsp. REDUCED CALORIE MAYONNAISE*
1/2 cup GREEN GRAPES
1 Tbsp. chopped PECANS**
1 Tbsp. PLAIN NONFAT YOGURT**
4 LETTUCE LEAVES

Combine apple, grapes, celery and pecans in a bowl; toss gently. Combine apple juice, yogurt and mayonnaise in a bowl, stirring with a wire whisk until smooth. Pour over apple mixture; toss well. Serve on lettuce-lined salad plates.

SERVING SIZE: 1/2 cup

CALORIES: 60    CHOL.: 1 mg.    FAT: 2.5 g. SODIUM: 39 mg.

\* = Dangerous to Some    \*\* = Consume with Caution    (see Pages 22 & 23)

# Jicama Salad

Quick and Easy—Prepare Ahead
**Makes 6 servings** **\*\*Green onions, yogurt, sour cream**

2 pkgs. (10 oz. each) frozen tiny GREEN PEAS, thawed
1 bunch GREEN ONIONS\*\*, chopped
1 Tbsp. REDUCED-FAT SOUR CREAM\*\*
1 cup chopped CELERY
3 cups BEAN SPROUTS, fresh or canned
1 cup PLAIN NONFAT YOGURT\*\*
1 JICAMA, peeled and chopped into 1-1/2 inch pieces
BLACK PEPPER

Drain peas well. Combine peas, bean sprouts, jicama, celery, green onions, yogurt, sour cream and pepper. Refrigerate until served.

SERVING SIZE: 1-1/4 cups

CALORIES: 152 CHOL.: 1 mg. FAT: 3 g. SODIUM: 161 mg.


# Mandarin Salad

Quick and Easy-—Prepare Ahead
**Makes 6 servings** **\*\*Mandarin oranges, onion**

2 cups HEAD LETTUCE, torn in pieces
1 cup chopped CELERY
1/2 tsp. SALT
3 Tbsp. WHITE VINEGAR
1 can (10-11 oz.) MANDARIN ORANGES\*\*, chilled

2 cups ROMAINE LETTUCE, torn in pieces
1 GREEN ONION\*\*, chopped
2 Tbsp. SUGAR
2 Tbsp. OLIVE OIL
dash TABASCO® SAUCE
dash PEPPER

Toss lettuce, celery and onion. Combine salt, pepper, sugar, vinegar, olive oil and Tabasco® sauce to make dressing. Drizzle 2 teaspoons dressing on lettuce. Top with Mandarin oranges.

Salad and dressing can be prepared separately ahead of time and refrigerated until ready to serve.

SERVING SIZE: 3/4 cup

CALORIES: 89 CHOL.: 0 FAT: 5 g. SODIUM: 4 mg.

\* = Dangerous to Some \*\* = Consume with Caution (see Pages 22 & 23)

# Strawberry-Banana Salad

Easy
Prepare Ahead
**Yogurt, banana

**Makes 9 servings**

*Be sure the banana is not over-ripe as the tyramine content, a blood pressure agent, increases with age.*

1-1/4 cup boiling WATER
1/2 cup LOW-FAT COTTAGE CHEESE
1/2 cup LOW-FAT STRAWBERRY-BANANA YOGURT**
1 large BANANA**, cut into 1 inch chunks (not too ripe)
1 envelope (.25 oz.) UNFLAVORED GELATIN
1 pkg. (3 oz.) SUGAR-FREE STRAWBERRY GELATIN
1 cup fresh WHOLE STRAWBERRIES, or unsweetened frozen

Place strawberry gelatin and the unflavored gelatin in a blender. Turn blender on low speed and slowly add boiling water. Blend until gelatins are dissolved. Turn blender up to medium speed and slowly add strawberries. Blend until smooth. Turn off blender and add remaining ingredients. Blend on medium speed until smooth and no cottage cheese particles can be seen.

Pour mixture into a 9-inch square pan. Refrigerate until set for 2 hours before serving. Cut into squares to serve.

NOTE: This recipe can be doubled and put into a mold. To serve as a dessert, pour the mixture into a graham cracker crumb pie crust and chill.

SERVING SIZE: 1/2 cup

CALORIES: 40    CHOL.: 1 mg.    FAT: 0.5 g.    SODIUM: 88 mg.

* = Dangerous to Some    ** = Consume with Caution    (see Pages 22 & 23)

# Taco Salad

**Easy**

Makes 6 servings     **\*\*Green onion, pinto beans**

*Fill pre-formed taco shells or, if you prefer the tortilla wedges, bake and serve separately. Add a long, cool beverage for a complete meal.*

1 pkg. (12 pieces) CORN TORTILLAS cut into wedges,
    or pre-formed and cooked TACO SHELLS
1-1/4 lbs. EXTRA LEAN GROUND BEEF
1 can (8-3/4 oz.) PINTO BEANS\*\*, drained and rinsed
1 GREEN PEPPER, seeded and chopped
2 GREEN ONIONS\*\*, diced, tops included
1 HEAD LETTUCE, leaves separated, washed,
    dried and torn
1 8-oz. jar CHUNKY SALSA
2 TOMATOES, cut into wedges
1 CUCUMBER, peeled and diced
8 BLACK OLIVES (optional)

Preheat oven to 350 degrees. Place tortillas on 2 flat baking sheets sprayed with non-stick product and sprinkle with salt, if desired, and bake 12 minutes. Turn them over and continue baking for an additional 5 minutes.

Brown meat in skillet or microwave oven. Drain well. Mix meat with 1 cup salsa and the pinto beans. Refrigerate.

Combine lettuce, tomato, cucumber, green pepper and green onion in bowl. Refrigerate. When ready to serve, combine lettuce mixture and meat mixture. Garnish with black olives, if desired. Serve with tortilla chips prepared as above or fill pre-formed taco shells. Use additional salsa as dressing.

SERVING SIZE: 1 cup of salad mixture, 2 corn tortillas

CALORIES: 397   CHOL.: 67 mg.   FAT: 13 g.   SODIUM: 247 mg.

* = Dangerous to Some   \*\* = Consume with Caution   (see Pages 22 & 23)

# Tuna and Brown Rice Salad

Quick and Easy
Prepare Ahead
**Lemon juice, sour cream

**Makes 4 servings**

*Substitute bulgar for the brown rice if you like. The rice (or bulgar) and peas have the right combination of amino acids to make a complete protein. There's plenty of that here!*

**1-1/4 cup (1/2 cup dry) cooked BROWN RICE**
**1 pkg. (10 oz.) frozen PEAS, thawed**
**1/2 cup shredded CARROT**
**1 tsp. PREPARED MUSTARD**
**1-1/2 tsp. LEMON JUICE****
**18 UNSALTED CRACKERS**
**1 can (6-1/2 oz.) SOLID-WHITE TUNA IN WATER, drained**
**1/2 cup LOWER-FAT SOUR CREAM****
**1/8 tsp. PEPPER**
**pinch SALT**
**LETTUCE LEAVES**

Mix together the rice, tuna, peas, sour cream, carrot, mustard, lemon juice, pepper and salt in a large bowl.

Arrange lettuce leaves on 4 plates. Using ice cream scoop, scoop about 1 cup tuna mixture on each plate of lettuce. Serve with 4 crackers each.

SERVING SIZE: 1 cup

CALORIES: 346   CHOL.: 26 mg.  FAT: 7 g.   SODIUM: 451 mg.

* = Dangerous to Some   ** = Consume with Caution   (see Pages 22 & 23)

# Tuna Pasta Salad a la Nicoise

**Quick and Easy**
**Prepare Ahead**
**\*Mayonnaise**
Makes about 6 servings      **\*\*Onion, lime peel, lime juice**

*A pasta variation for tuna salad; the red onions and green beans add color and crunch.*

1 cup REDUCED CALORIE MAYONNAISE\* (check label)
1 tsp. grated LIME PEEL\*\*
2 cups (4-1/2 oz.) SEA SHELL MACARONI, cooked and
    drained
1 pkg. (9 oz.) frozen cut GREEN BEANS, cooked,
    drained and chilled
2 Tbsp. LIME JUICE\*\*
1/2 tsp. DRIED TARRAGON
1/2 cup coarsely chopped RED ONION\*\*
1 can (6-1/2 oz.) WATER-PACKED TUNA, drained and flaked
6 LETTUCE LEAVES

In large bowl stir mayonnaise, lime juice, grated lime peel and tarragon until smooth.  Add macaroni, green beans, tuna and onion.  Cover; chill at least 2 hours to blend flavors.  Arrange on lettuce-lined platter.  Garnish with tomatoes and serve with a cup of hot *Creamy Romano Tomato Soup* (see *Soups*)

SERVING SIZE: 1 cup

CALORIES: 250   CHOL.: 5 mg.  FAT: 9 g.  SODIUM: 290 mg.

\* = Dangerous to Some    \*\* = Consume with Caution   (see Pages 22 & 23)

# Spanish Potato Salad

**Makes 10 servings**

*A hot potato salad that can be made ahead of time and reheated for a party, where it will be a favorite with everyone. Always taste before serving and adjust seasonings.*

1/4 cup **MARGARINE**
1/4 cup **WHITE VINEGAR**
1/4 tsp. **GROUND BLACK PEPPER**
1/3 cup finely chopped **ONION****
8 medium **POTATOES**, peeled, diced and cooked.
1 Tbsp. **SUGAR**
1/4 tsp. **DRY MUSTARD**
1/3 cup finely chopped **GREEN PEPPER**
1/4 cup diced **PIMENTOS**

Melt margarine and combine with vinegar, sugar, pepper and dry mustard. Mix in green pepper, onion and pimento pieces. Pour over drained warm potatoes and serve immediately.

SERVING SIZE: 3/4 cup

CALORIES: 103   CHOL.: 0      FAT: 5.g.   SODIUM: 43 mg.

* = Dangerous to Some   ** = Consume with Caution   (see Pages 22 & 23)

# Catalina Salad Dressing

**Quick and Easy**
**Prepare Ahead**
**Makes 4 cups**                    **\*\*Lemon Juice, Onion**

*A make-ahead low-calorie dressing for mixed greens or salads or a zesty addition for lean cuts of meat and poultry.*

**3-1/2 cups (28 oz. can) crushed TOMATOES**
**1/3 cup sliced SHALLOTS\*\***
**1/4 cup finely chopped PARSLEY**
**1 tsp. dried OREGANO LEAVES, crushed**
**1/2 tsp. DRY MUSTARD**
**1/4 tsp. BLACK PEPPER**
**1/2 cup finely chopped GREEN PEPPER**
**1/3 cup WHITE VINEGAR**
**3 Tbsp. fresh LEMON JUICE\*\***
**1 tsp. GARLIC SALT**
**1/2 tsp. DRIED TARRAGON LEAVES, crushed**

In large bowl, blend crushed tomatoes, green pepper, shallots, vinegar, parsley, lemon juice, oregano, garlic salt, tarragon, dry mustard and black pepper. Cover, refrigerate for 3 to 4 hours to allow flavors to blend. Serve over salad greens.

SERVING SIZE: 2 tablespoons

CALORIES: 18     CHOL.: 0     FAT: 0     SODIUM: 260 mg.

---

* = Dangerous to Some     ** = Consume with Caution     (see Pages 22 & 23)

# Creamy (Blender) Mayonnaise

Quick and Easy
Prepare Ahead
**Onion powder

**Makes 1-1/2 cups**

*Homemade mayonnaise has an appeal over commercial and you have control over the ingredients! If your mayonnaise starts to separate, add more of the combining agent, egg.*

| | |
|---|---|
| 1/3 cup EGG SUBSTITUTE | 1 tsp. DRY MUSTARD |
| 1/4 tsp. ONION POWDER** | 1/2 tsp. PAPRIKA |
| dash GROUND RED PEPPER | 2 Tbsp. WHITE VINEGAR |
| 1 cup VEGETABLE OIL | |

Combine all ingredients and 1/2 cup oil in a blender container. Cover and blend on medium-high speed just until mixed. Without turning blender off, very slowly pour in other 1/2 cup oil in a fine steady stream. If necessary, use rubber spatula to keep mixture flowing to blades. Continue blending until oil is completely incorporated and mixture is smooth and thick. Store in refrigerator.

SERVING SIZE: 1 tablespoon

CALORIES: 45    CHOL.: 0    FAT: 5 g.    SODIUM: 4 mg.

# Basic Italian Dressing

Quick and Easy
Prepare Ahead

**Makes 1-1/2 cups**

| | |
|---|---|
| 1 cup VEGETABLE OIL | BASIL LEAVES |
| 2 tsp. SUGAR | TARRAGON LEAVES |
| 1 cup WHITE VINEGAR | DILL WEED or OREGANO |
| DRY MUSTARD | LEAVES |

Combine oil, vinegar and sugar in jar with tight-fitting lid and shake vigorously. Season to taste with dry mustard, tarragon, basil, dill or oregano.

SERVING SIZE: 1 tablespoon

CALORIES: 82    CHOL.: 0    FAT: 9 g.    SODIUM: 0

* = Dangerous to Some    ** = Consume with Caution    (see Pages 22 & 23)

# Cucumber Dressing

**Makes 1-3/4 cups**

**Quick and Easy**
**\*\*Lemon juice, onion**

*This can be used as a substitute for tartar sauce with fish or on baked potatoes for a reduced-calorie topping.*

**1 cup 1% LOW-FAT COTTAGE CHEESE**
**2 Tbsp. chopped fresh PARSLEY**
**1 Tbsp. LEMON JUICE\*\***
**1/2 cup seeded, diced, unpeeled CUCUMBER**
**1/4 cup SKIM MILK**
**2 Tbsp. sliced GREEN ONIONS\*\***
**1-1/2 tsp. PREPARED HORSERADISH**

Combine cottage cheese, skim milk, parsley, onions, lemon juice and horseradish in the container of an electric blender; cover and process until smooth. Add cucumber, process just until coarsely chopped. Serve over lettuce wedges.

SERVING SIZE: 1 tablespoon

CALORIES: 7    CHOL.: 0    FAT: 0.1 g.    SODIUM: 34 mg.


# Sprout Dressing

**Makes 2 cups**

**Quick and Easy**
**\*\*Lemon juice**

*If you want to put variety into your salads, try preparing this healthy and tasty dressing.*

**1-1/2 cups ALFALFA or RADISH SPROUTS**
**1/2 cup VEGETABLE OIL**
**2 Tbsp. LEMON JUICE\*\* or WHITE VINEGAR**
**1/2 tsp. PREPARED MUSTARD**
**SALT and PEPPER to taste**

Combine all ingredients in blender. Blend until smooth, about 1 minute. Serve on salad or use as fruit or vegetable dip.

SERVING SIZE: 1 tablespoon

CALORIES: 86    CHOL.: 0    FAT: 9 g.    SODIUM: 1 mg.


\* = Dangerous to Some    \*\* = Consume with Caution    (see Pages 22 & 23)

# Egg Salad Dressing

**Makes 1/2 cup**

Quick and Easy
**Lemon juice

*The eggs add a satisfying but low-calorie richness to this dressing.*

3 hard-cooked EGGS or 3/4 cup EGG SUBSTITUTE, cooked
2 tsp. LEMON JUICE**
2 Tbsp. WATER
1 Tbsp. WHITE VINEGAR
SALT and PEPPER to taste
GARLIC POWDER to taste

Put eggs in blender and blend. Add water, vinegar and lemon juice. Add salt and pepper and garlic powder to taste. Blend until mixture is creamy.

SERVING SIZE: 1 tablespoon

CALORIES: 41   CHOL.: 137 mg.  FAT: 3 g.  SODIUM: 35 mg.

# Flavorful French Dressing

**Makes approximately 1 pint**

Quick and Easy
**Onion

*This quickly assembled salad dressing is a great favorite with everyone. Tasty with both vegetable and fruit salads.*

1/2 cup SALAD OIL
1/2 cup WHITE VINEGAR
1 tsp. SALT
1 Tbsp. grated ONION**, or 1 Tbsp. minced
    dehydrated onion**
1/2 cup SUGAR
1/4 cup CATSUP
1 tsp. PAPRIKA

Combine above ingredients in large jar (you may prefer to make a one-half recipe). Shake well before serving.

SERVING SIZE: 1 tablespoon

CALORIES: 67   CHOL.: 0   FAT: 6.4 g.  SODIUM: 214 mg.

* = Dangerous to Some   ** = Consume with Caution   (see Pages 22 & 23)

# Vegetable Entrées

# Cajun Rice

**Quick and Easy—Prepare Ahead**

Makes 8 servings                                          **\*\*Onion**

1-1/4 cups WATER
1/2 tsp. HOT PEPPER SAUCE
1 cup uncooked REGULAR RICE
1 can (14-1/2 oz.) STEWED TOMATOES, undrained
2 Tbsp. OIL
1 large ONION\*\*, chopped
1 Tbsp. minced GARLIC
1 large GREEN PEPPER, chopped

In medium skillet, heat oil over medium-high heat. Stir in rice, onion, pepper and garlic. Sauté 3 minutes. Stir in tomatoes, water and hot pepper sauce, breaking tomatoes with a spoon. Bring to a boil; reduce heat; cover and simmer, stirring occasionally, 20 minutes or until liquid is absorbed and rice is tender.

SERVING SIZE: 3/4 cup

CALORIES: 140     CHOL.: 0     FAT: 4 g.     SODIUM: 135 mg.

# Linguine with Tomato Sauce

**Quick and Easy—Prepare Ahead**

Makes 4 servings

1-1/2 lbs. ripe ROMAN TOMATOES coarsely chopped
2 Tbsp. VEGETABLE OIL
2 cups loosely packed fresh BASIL, chopped, or 2 cups
    chopped PARSLEY plus 1 Tbsp. dried BASIL
2 Tbsp. WHITE VINEGAR
3 CLOVES GARLIC, minced or pressed
8 oz. LINGUINE, cooked and drained

In large skillet heat oil over medium-high heat. Add garlic; sauté 1 minute. Stir in tomatoes, bring to boil. Reduce heat; cover; simmer 5 minutes, stirring occasionally, or until sauce thickens slightly, stir in basil and vinegar. Serve with linguine.

SERVING SIZE: 2/3 cup

CALORIES: 320     CHOL.: 0          FAT: 8 g.     SODIUM: 25 mg.

\* = Dangerous to Some     \*\* = Consume with Caution     (see Pages 22 & 23)

# Carrot-Broccoli-Mushroom Stir Fry

**Quick and Easy**
***Mushrooms**
****Onion, lemon juice**

**Makes 8 servings**

*Stir fry originated because of the Oriental shortage of fuels. The result was many small, quickly cooked, but not overly-cooked, ingredients.*

3/4 lb. MUSHROOMS*, sliced thin
3 medium GREEN ONIONS**
1 Tbsp. MARGARINE
1 tsp. LEMON JUICE**
2 Tbsp. WHITE VINEGAR
1 lb. fresh BROCCOLI
1 lb. CARROTS, peeled and thinly sliced
1 Tbsp. VEGETABLE OIL
1 tsp. NUTMEG
1 tsp. THYME
Freshly ground BLACK PEPPER

Wash broccoli, peel stems and cut into 2-inch lengths. Separate broccoli florets by cutting into quarters so they are of uniform size.

In a large skillet or wok, heat margarine and oil over medium heat. Add broccoli, carrots, mushrooms and onions. Cook and stir until vegetables are tender-crisp, about 5 minutes. Stir in lemon juice, vinegar and other seasonings and serve immediately.

SERVING SIZE: 2/3 cup

CALORIES: 93    CHOL.: 0    FAT: 3.7 g.    SODIUM: 61.6 mg

* = Dangerous to Some    ** = Consume with Caution    (see Pages 22 & 23)

# Green Bean & Rice Casserole

**Quick and Easy—Prepare Ahead**
***Mushrooms**

**Makes 6 servings**                                     ****Onion**

*A casserole that is easy to make and is an economical taste treat. The beans and rice combination serve as a complete protein replacement for meat.*

**1 can (10-3/4 oz.) condensed CREAM OF MUSHROOM soup***
**1/2 cup SKIM MILK**
**1/2 tsp. DRIED MARJORAM**
**1/8 tsp. PEPPER**
**PAPRIKA**
**1 pkg. (9 oz.) frozen FRENCH-STYLE GREEN BEANS,**
    **cooked and drained**
**1/4 cup sliced GREEN ONIONS****
**1/4 tsp. GARLIC POWDER**
**3 cups COOKED RICE, unsalted**

In 1-1/2-quart casserole, combine soup, milk, marjoram, garlic powder and pepper. Stir in beans, green onions and rice. Cover, bake at 350 degrees for 25 minutes or until hot and bubbling. Sprinkle with paprika. Bake uncovered 5 minutes more.

MICROWAVE: In large bowl, combine soup, milk, marjoram, garlic powder and pepper. Stir in beans, green onions and rice. Spread rice mixture evenly in a 12 x 8-inch microwave-proof baking dish. Cover with vented plastic wrap; microwave on HIGH (100% power) 10 minutes or until edges are bubbling and center is hot, rotating dish once halfway through heating. Sprinkle with paprika. Microwave uncovered 1 minute.

SERVING SIZE: 2/3 cup

**Recipe**
CALORIES: 174   CHOL.: 4 mg.   FAT: 4 g.   SODIUM: 325 mg.

**From Soup**
CALORIES: 44   CHOL.: 1 mg.   FAT: 3 g.   SODIUM: 237 mg.

* = Dangerous to Some   ** = Consume with Caution   (see Pages 22 & 23)

# Mediterranean Vegetables

**Quick and Easy**
**Prepare Ahead**
**\*\*Onion**

**Makes 4 servings**

*This Middle Eastern entrée features eggplant, so popular in that part of the world. Add the touch of thyme for pizzazz.*

**1-1/2 cups sliced ONIONS\*\***
**1-1/2 cups thickly sliced ZUCCHINI**
**1/2 tsp. crushed fresh GARLIC**
**1/4 tsp. THYME leaves**
**1 can (16 oz.) LOW-SODIUM TOMATOES, coarsely chopped**
**1 Tbsp. MARGARINE**
**1 cup GREEN PEPPER strips**
**2 cups cubed unpeeled EGGPLANT**
**1 BAY LEAF**
**dash GROUND BLACK PEPPER**

Melt margarine in a large heavy pan over medium heat. Add onions, green pepper and garlic; sauté, stirring occasionally, until onions are transparent, about 5 minutes. Mix in tomatoes, eggplant, zucchini, thyme, bay leaf and pepper. Cover and simmer over medium-low heat, stirring occasionally, until vegetables are tender, about 15 minutes. Remove cover and cook an additional 5 to 10 minutes. Remove bay leaf.

MICROWAVE: In 3-quart microwave-proof casserole, combine all ingredients except tomatoes. Cover, microwave on HIGH (100% power) for 8 minutes. Stir in tomatoes; cover; microwave on HIGH for 5 to 7 minutes.

SERVING SIZE: 1-1/2 cups

CALORIES: 93     CHOL.: 0     FAT: 3 g.     SODIUM: 44 mg.

---

\* = Dangerous to Some    \*\* = Consume with Caution    (see Pages 22 & 23)

# Mexicali Rice

**Makes 6 servings**

*Spanish rice didn't become famous for nothing. Make this as hot as you like via the hot pepper sauce.*

2-1/4 cups WATER
1/2 cup chopped ONION**
1/4 tsp. crushed fresh GARLIC
1 cup uncooked LONG GRAIN RICE
1/2 cup (4 cubes) frozen *LOW-SODIUM TOMATO BASE*,
  or *TOMATO FRESH SALSA* (see *Sauces*)
2 Tbsp. MARGARINE
1/4 cup chopped GREEN PEPPER
1/4 tsp. OREGANO LEAVES
1/8 tsp. GROUND BLACK PEPPER
3-4 drops HOT PEPPER SAUCE

In large skillet, melt margarine over medium heat. Stir in onion, green pepper and garlic; sauté until tender, stirring occasionally, 2 to 2-1/2 minutes. Stir in rice; cook and stir until golden, about 1-1/2 to 2 minutes. Add water, tomato base, oregano, pepper and hot pepper sauce. Cook and stir until tomato base melts. Reduce heat to low; cover and cook until rice is tender and liquid is absorbed, 20 to 25 minutes. Fluff rice with fork and serve hot.

MICROWAVE:  IN 2-quart microwave-proof casserole, melt margarine on HIGH (100% power) for 40 to 45 seconds. Add onion and garlic; microwave on HIGH for 2 minutes, stirring after 1 minute. Stir in water, tomato base, oregano, pepper and hot pepper sauce. Cover; microwave on HIGH for 18 to 20 minutes, stirring after 9 minutes. Let stand 2 to 3 minutes; stir before serving.

SERVING SIZE: 2/3 cup

CALORIES: 167   CHOL.: 0   FAT: 4 g.   SODIUM: 41 mg.

* = Dangerous to Some   ** = Consume with Caution   (see Pages 22 & 23)

# Ratatouille

**Makes 4 servings**

*Simple proof that lack of fat need not compromise flavor.
Eggplant easily picks up the flavor of the other ingredients.
Serve with rice and very lean ground beef.*

1 small sweet GREEN PEPPER
1 tsp. VEGETABLE OIL
1 medium-size ripe TOMATO
1 small EGGPLANT (3/4 lb.)
2 Tbsp. minced fresh PARSLEY leaves
1 medium-size ONION**
1 GARLIC CLOVE, minced
1 medium-size ZUCCHINI (1/2 lb.)
1/2 tsp. DRIED BASIL
1/2 tsp. DRIED THYME

Cut the green pepper into strips. Slice the onion. Sauté pepper and onion in oil. Chop the tomato and slice the zucchini into 1/4-inch-thick slices. Cube the eggplant; add the tomato, zucchini, eggplant, garlic, basil, thyme and parsley to the pepper and onion mixture. Simmer until the vegetables are tender.

SERVING SIZE: 3/4 cup

CALORIES: 47    CHOL.: 0    FAT: 2 g.    SODIUM: 7 mg.

* = Dangerous to Some    ** = Consume with Caution    (see Pages 22 & 23)

# Red Chile Linguine

**Quick and Easy—Prepare ahead**
**Makes 6 servings**                                    **\*\*Lime juice**

*The traditional linguine comes with more than its share of saturated fat.*

1/4 cup OLIVE OIL                    1 LIME\*\*, juiced
1/2 tsp. RED PEPPER FLAKES           8 oz. LINGUINE,
1/4 cup PARSLEY, chopped                 cooked
2 tsp. GARLIC, minced

Heat olive oil in skillet; add garlic; sauté 1 minute. Add red pepper, sauté 30 seconds. Add cooked linguine; stir well and cook over medium heat until hot and well coated. Add parsley, stir well; add lime juice. Toss well and serve.

SERVING SIZE: 2/3 cup

CALORIES: 364    CHOL.: 0    FAT: 10 g.    SODIUM: 8 mg.

# Rice-Stuffed Squash

**Easy**
**Makes 4 servings**      **\*\*Orange rind, orange juice, walnuts**

*Very flavorful because of the contrast of crunchy walnuts, squash and orange.*

2 medium-size ACORN SQUASH       1/2 cup RICE, cooked
1 tsps. grated ORANGE RIND\*\*      1/2 cup chopped
1-2 Tbsp. frozen ORANGE JUICE         WALNUTS\*\*
    CONCENTRATE\*\*

Cut the squash in half and remove the seeds. Combine the remaining ingredients and fill the squash with the mixture. Place in a baking pan; cover with aluminum foil or lid and bake in 400 degree oven for about 35 minutes, or until squash is fork-tender. Extra orange juice concentrate can be drizzled over the squash just before serving.

SERVING SIZE: 1/2 squash

CALORIES:  204   CHOL.: 0      FAT: 10 g. SODIUM: 20 mg.

* = Dangerous to Some   ** = Consume with Caution   (see Pages 22 & 23)

# Spaghetti Squash 'n Sauce

**Quick and Easy**
**Makes 4 servings**

*An inexpensive main dish, easy to fix and colorful, for spaghetti squash devotees. Increase the cottage cheese on the side for protein.*

**1 YELLOW SPAGHETTI SQUASH**
**1 jar (32 oz.) bottled SPAGHETTI SAUCE**
**4 tsp. COTTAGE CHEESE**

Preheat oven to 350 degrees. Poke spaghetti squash several times with long fork. Place on baking sheet. Bake for 1 hour. Cut squash in half and remove seeds. Pull spaghetti strands free with a fork. Heat spaghetti sauce. For each serving, ladle 1 cup sauce onto 2 cups spaghetti squash. Top with 1 teaspoon cottage cheese.

MICROWAVE: Poke spaghetti squash several times with long fork. Place in microwave-safe baking dish. Microwave on HIGH (100% power) 4 to 6 minutes. Turn squash over and microwave for another 4 to 6 minutes. Remove from oven and let stand 5 to 10 minutes. Cut squash in half and remove seeds. Pull spaghetti squash strands free with a fork. Place squash in baking dish; ladle sauce over squash; return to microwave and heat through. Sprinkle with cottage cheese. Serve with **Applesauce Spice Muffins** (see *Breads*) and **Strawberry-Banana Salad** (see *Salads*).

SERVING SIZE: 1 cup spaghetti squash with 1 cup of sauce

CALORIES: 287    chol.: 1 mg.    FAT: 12 g.    SODIUM: 324 mg.

* = Dangerous to Some    ** = Consume with Caution    (see Pages 22 & 23)

# Spaghetti with Bean Sauce

**Makes 10 servings**

Prepare Ahead
*Pinto & kidney beans
**Onion

*This entrée equals a meat dish because of the combination of beans and a grain (the wheat-based spaghetti).*

1 medium ONION**, chopped
2 Tbsp. VEGETABLE OIL
1-1/2 cups dried PINTO* or KIDNEY BEANS*, washed
1/2 tsp. PEPPER
1/4 tsp. crumbled DRIED BASIL
1/4 tsp. crumbled DRIED OREGANO
2 BEEF BOUILLON CUBES
1 CLOVE GARLIC, minced
1 dried HOT PEPPER, crumbled
1 tsp. SALT
1 Tbsp. WHITE VINEGAR
4 cups WATER
1 can (16 oz.) TOMATOES
1 can (6 oz.) TOMATO PASTE
SPAGHETTI

Sauté onion and garlic in oil for 5 minutes. Add beans, hot pepper, salt, pepper and water. Cover and simmer for 30 minutes. Add remaining ingredients and simmer, uncovered, for about 1 hour, stirring occasionally. Serve sauce over cooked spaghetti, macaroni or noodles.

**Pasta:**
SERVING SIZE: 1/2 cup

CALORIES: 100    CHOL.: 0    FAT: 0    SODIUM: 1 mg.

**Sauce:**
SERVING SIZE: 3/4 cup

CALORIES: 165    CHOL.: 0    FAT: 3 g.    SODIUM: 1 mg.

* = Dangerous to Some    ** = Consume with Caution    (see Pages 22 & 23)

# Spinach Pie

Specialty
**Onion

**Makes 4 servings**

*This recipe can also be served as an appetizer.*

**The crust: (or use prepared crust)**

3/4 cup ALL-PURPOSE FLOUR

3 Tbsp. REDUCED-CALORIE MARGARINE

1/8 tsp. SALT

2 Tbsp. ICE WATER

Combine flour and salt in medium-size bowl. Work in margarine with fork or pastry blender until mixture is crumbly. Add water and work until dough is formed. Pat dough into a disk. Place between 2 sheets waxed paper. Roll out into 11-inch circle. Fit into 7-1/2 inch fluted tart pan with removable bottom. Place square of aluminum foil in crust; add dried beans or rice to weight crust. Bake in preheated very hot oven (450 degrees) for 5 minutes. Remove foil and beans. Bake crust 10 minutes longer or until lightly browned. Remove from oven. Lower oven temperature to moderate (375 degrees).

**The filling:**

1/2 cup LOW-FAT (1%) MILK

1 pkg. (10 oz.) chopped FROZEN SPINACH, thawed and drained well

1/4 tsp. BLACK PEPPER

1/4 cup chopped ONION**

1 CLOVE GARLIC, finely chopped

2 EGGS, beaten slightly

1/8 tsp. SALT

Spray 10-inch nonstick skillet with vegetable cooking spray. Add onion and garlic and sauté over medium heat for 2 minutes. Squeeze out excess liquid from spinach with paper toweling. Add spinach to skillet; cook 1 minute; remove to medium-size bowl. Add milk, eggs, salt and pepper to spinach mixture; stir to combine; pour into crust.

Bake in preheated moderate oven (375 degrees) for 30 to 35 minutes or until center is set. Let stand about 10 minutes. Remove sides from pan. Cut pie into wedges to serve.

SERVING SIZE: 1/4 pie

CALORIES: 200   CHOL.: 145 mg.   FAT: 9 g.   SODIUM: 372 mg.

* = Dangerous to Some   ** = Consume with Caution   (see Pages 22 & 23)

# Spinach Potpourri

**Quick and Easy**
***Mushrooms**
****Onion, yogurt**

**Makes 6 servings**

*A very complete meal low in fat but high in flavor and nutrition. The combination of onion, mushroom soup, potatoes and spinach can be ready in half an hour if planned ahead.*

**1/4 cup chopped RED ONION****
**1/8 tsp. GROUND NUTMEG**
**1 can (10-3/4 oz.) condensed CREAM OF MUSHROOM SOUP***
**1 soup can plus 2 Tbsp. WATER**
**1/2 cup SKIM MILK**
**1 pkg. (10 oz.) frozen chopped SPINACH**
**1-1/2 cups peeled, diced cooked POTATOES**
**1/8 tsp. PEPPER**
**1/2 cup PLAIN NONFAT YOGURT****

In 2-quart covered saucepan, over high heat, cook onion, spinach and 2 tablespoons of the water 10 minutes or until vegetables are tender, stirring occasionally.

Reduce heat to medium. Blend in soup, remaining soup can of water, nutmeg and pepper. Cover; simmer 10 minutes. Stir in yogurt and potatoes. Heat through. DO NOT BOIL.

SERVING SIZE: 1 cup

**Recipe**
CALORIES: 98    CHOL.: 1 mg.    FAT: 3 g.    SODIUM: 307 mg.

**From Soup**
CALORIES: 44    CHOL.: 1 mg.    FAT: 3 g.    SODIUM: 237 mg.

* = Dangerous to Some    ** = Consume with Caution    (see Pages 22 & 23)

# Vegetable Medley Quiche

**Specialty**
**Makes 8 servings**

*Everyone seems to like quiche; this one sings with color, as well as flavor and nutrition.*

1 small ZUCCHINI, sliced (about 1 cup)
1/4 tsp. BASIL LEAVES
1 small GREEN PEPPER, cut in strips (about 3/4 cup)
1 (8 oz.) carton EGG SUBSTITUTE, or 4 EGGS
1 tsp. MARGARINE
1 cup SKIM MILK
1 (9 inch) PASTRY CRUST
1 small RED PEPPER, cut in strips (about 3/4 cup)
1/8 tsp. GROUND BLACK PEPPER

In skillet, over medium heat, cook zucchini, green pepper and red pepper in margarine until tender crisp, stirring occasionally. Spoon mixture into pastry crust. Mix egg substitute, skim milk, basil and pepper; pour over vegetables. Bake at 375 degrees for 50 to 55 minutes or until knife inserted in center comes out clean. Let stand 10 minutes before serving. Serve with a small side salad and a square of ***Honey Walnut Cake*** (see *Desserts*).

SERVING SIZE: 1/8 pie wedge

CALORIES: 127   CHOL.: 13 mg.  FAT: 8 g.  SODIUM: 211 mg.

* = Dangerous to Some   ** = Consume with Caution   (see Pages 22 & 23)

# Vegetable Platter with Mustard Sauce

**Makes 8 servings**

*This dish focuses on two anti-cancer, cruciferous ingredients.*

1 pkg. (10 oz.) frozen BRUSSEL SPROUTS
1/2 sweet RED PEPPER, cut into 2-inch julienne strips
1/2 cup SKIM MILK
1 small CAULIFLOWER, washed and trimmed
    but not cut up
1 Tbsp. FLOUR
1 Tbsp. DIJON MUSTARD
dash WHITE PEPPER

In large saucepan, over medium-high heat, steam whole cauliflower head in 1-inch of water 12 to 15 minutes or until tender. Remove to platter and keep warm. Cook Brussel sprouts according to package directions. In small saucepan, over medium heat, combine flour, milk, mustard and pepper. Cook 5 minutes or until sauce thickens, stirring constantly. Arrange Brussel sprouts around cauliflower head on serving platter, with pepper strips between Brussel sprouts. Pour sauce over cauliflower head.

MICROWAVE: On a microwave-safe serving platter, arrange cauliflower head upside down in center of platter. Arrange Brussel sprouts around cauliflower. Cover entire platter with plastic wrap. Microwave 3 minutes on HIGH (100% power). Uncover platter, turn cauliflower right side up and re-cover with plastic wrap. Microwave 4-1/2 to 5 minutes more or until cauliflower and sprouts are tender. Let stand while preparing sauce. In 4-cup microwave-safe bowl, combine flour, milk, mustard and pepper. Microwave on HIGH 1 to 1-1/2 minutes or until mixture thickens, stirring halfway through cooking. Uncover vegetables. Garnish with red pepper strips and top with mustard sauce. Serve with *Date-Nut Bread* (see *Breads*) and *Caramel Custard* (see *Desserts*).

SERVING SIZE: 3/4 cup

CALORIES: 35    CHOL.: 1 mg.    FAT: 1 g.    SODIUM: 50 mg.

\* = Dangerous to Some   ** = Consume with Caution   (see Pages 22 & 23)

# Meat Entrées

# Apple Stuffed Veal Rolls

**Makes 4 servings**

*Your grandmother prepared veal in a similar way with bread stuffing and called the dish "veal birds".*

1/2 cup chopped onion**
3 cups day-old WHITE BREAD cubes
1/2 cup WATER
1 lb. thinly sliced VEAL CUTLETS (4 large slices)
1/2 cup diagonally sliced CELERY, blanched
2 Tbsp. MARGARINE
1 cup diced APPLE
1 cup APPLE JUICE
1 Tbsp. CORNSTARCH
dash GROUND BLACK PEPPER
1/2 cup APPLE slices, blanched

Sauté onion in 1 tablespoon margarine until golden, about 5 minutes. Stir in bread cubes. Heat, stirring until margarine is absorbed. Stir in diced apple, pepper and 1/4 cup water.

Place 1/4 stuffing mixture (about 1/2 cup) near one edge of each cutlet. Roll up cutlets like a jelly roll. Melt remaining margarine in skillet over medium heat. Brown veal rolls on all sides. Add 1 cup apple juice to skillet. Cover and cook until veal is tender, about 15 to 20 minutes. Remove veal rolls to a warm platter.

Mix together remaining 1/4 cup water and cornstarch. Stir into pan juices. Cook until thickened, stirring constantly. Spoon over veal rolls and garnish platter with blanched celery and apple slices. Serve with **Harlequin Slaw** (see *Salads*), whole wheat bread and **Cannoli Cream** (see *Desserts*).

SERVING SIZE: 1 veal roll

CALORIES: 388   CHOL.: 82 mg.  FAT: 16 g. SODIUM: 312 mg.

* = Dangerous to Some   ** = Consume with Caution   (see Pages 22 & 23)

# Barbecue Pork on a Bun

Quick and Easy
Prepare Ahead
*Pork

**Makes 4 servings**          **Onion, orange juice, oranges

*Now that pork is so much leaner, some nutritionists refer to pork as "another white meat".*

1 large ONION**, finely chopped
1 can (8 oz.) no-salt added or regular TOMATO SAUCE
1-2 Tbsp. WHITE VINEGAR
2 tsp. PREPARED MUSTARD
2 cups cooked SHREDDED PORK*
4 HAMBURGER BUNS, split and toasted
NON-STICK VEGETABLE COOKING OIL
2 Tbsp. LIGHT BROWN SUGAR
1 Tbsp. ORANGE JUICE**
1/8 tsp. PAPRIKA
1/8 tsp. GROUND HOT RED PEPPER
2 juice ORANGES**, cut into wedges

Spray medium size non-stick saucepan with cooking spray. Sauté onion in saucepan for 2 minutes or until tender. (Add a little water if necessary to prevent sticking.) Stir in tomato sauce, sugar, vinegar, orange juice, mustard, paprika and red pepper. Bring to boiling. Lower heat; simmer, covered 5 to 8 minutes or until thickened. Stir in pork.

To serve, spoon meat and sauce over toasted bun. Garnish with orange wedges and serve with *Mandarin Salad* (see *Salads*) and a *Saucepan Butterscotch Brownie* (see *Desserts*).

SERVING SIZE: 1/2 cup per bun

CALORIES: 315   CHOL.: 58 mg.  FAT: 5 g.  SODIUM: 292 mg.

* = Dangerous to Some   ** = Consume with Caution   (see Pages 22 & 23)

# Beef Cubed Steaks

**Quick and Easy**
**Makes 2 servings**

*Vegetable and cube steaks can be ready to eat in less time than it takes to eat them.*

1 CLOVE GARLIC, minced
2 lean BEEF CUBED STEAKS (about 4 oz. each)
1 tsp. OLIVE OIL
2 small ZUCCHINI, thinly sliced, or 10 oz. frozen BROCCOLI
1/2 tsp. dried BASIL LEAVES
1/4 tsp. PEPPER
1/4 tsp. SALT
4 CHERRY TOMATOES, halved

Combine garlic, basil and pepper; divide seasoning mixture in half. Press half of seasoning mixture evenly into both sides of beef cubed steaks; set aside.

Heat oil and remaining seasoning mixture in large non-stick frying pan over medium heat. Add zucchini or broccoli; cook and stir 2 to 3 minutes. Add tomatoes and cook 1 minute. Remove vegetables to warm platter and keep warm.

Increase heat to medium-high; add steaks, cook steaks 3 to 4 minutes, turning once. Season steaks with salt. Serve with vegetables, relishes, **Low-Salt Challa Bread** (see *Breads*), **Broccoli Pasta Salad** (see *Salads*), and **Baked Apple Crumble** (see *Desserts*).

SERVING SIZE: 1 steak and 1/2 of vegetables

CALORIES: 279   CHOL.: 77 mg.  FAT: 15 g. SODIUM: 670 mg.

* = Dangerous to Some   ** = Consume with Caution   (see Pages 22 & 23)

# Beef Picadillo

**Makes 6 servings**

*Add variety to your meal plans by preparing an ethnic dish that is both tasty and healthy.*

1-1/2 lbs. trimmed ROUND STEAK, cut into thin strips
1/2 tsp. DRIED OREGANO LEAVES
1/8 tsp. GARLIC POWDER
1 Tbsp. MARGARINE
1 TOMATO, chopped
1 jar (12 oz.) SALSA, mild, medium or hot
2 Tbsp. instant, minced or chopped ONION**

In large skillet, over medium-high heat, cook round steak strips in margarine about 5 minutes or until meat is no longer pink. Stir in salsa, tomato, oregano, onion and garlic powder. Simmer for 10 minutes, stirring occasionally.

MICROWAVE: Melt margarine in microwave-safe dish. Mix round steak strips with margarine. Cover dish. Cook on HIGH (100% power) for 2 to 3 minutes or until meat is no longer pink. Stir after 1 to 1-1/2 minutes. Stir in salsa, tomato, oregano, onion and garlic powder. Cook for 3 to 4 minutes on HIGH, stirring occasionally.

Serve with **Roasted Garlic Potatoes** (see *Side Dishes*) and a tossed salad with **Sprout Dressing** *(see Salads)*.

SERVING SIZE: 3/4 cup

CALORIES: 202   CHOL.: 70 mg.  FAT: 9 g.  SODIUM: 215 mg.

* = Dangerous to Some   ** = Consume with Caution   (see Pages 22 & 23)

# Cajun Jambalaya

**Makes 5 servings**

Specialty
Prepare Ahead
**Onion

*Louisiana contributes this complete meal for a change from the ordinary casserole. Caution: You may want to start with less than 1/4 teaspoon of cayenne pepper! You can always add more, but wait a moment to see.*

1 Tbsp. VEGETABLE OIL
1/2 cup chopped CELERY
1 can (16 oz.) WHOLE TOMATOES with juice
1/2 cup LONG GRAIN RICE
1/4 tsp. CAYENNE PEPPER
1/8 tsp. GROUND THYME
1-1/2 cups chopped, cooked CHICKEN (skin and
        fat removed)
1/2 cup chopped ONIONS**
1 cup FAT-FREE CHICKEN BROTH
1/2 cup chopped GREEN PEPPER
1/2 tsp. SALT
1 Tbsp. chopped PARSLEY
1/2 cup chopped, cooked LEAN BEEF

Preheat a 2-quart saucepan over medium heat. Add oil, onions, peppers and celery. Cook, stirring frequently over medium heat until the onions are soft but not browned. Add tomatoes and juice, broth, rice, salt, pepper, parsley and thyme to the vegetables. Cook uncovered 20-25 minutes, stirring frequently, until rice is cooked. If the mixture gets too dry, add hot water. Add chicken and lean beef and continue to cook until heated through. Serve hot.

SERVING SIZE: 1 cup

CALORIES: 224   CHOL.: 87 mg.  FAT: 23 g. SODIUM: 551 mg.

* = Dangerous to Some   ** = Consume with Caution   (see Pages 22 & 23)

# Chili Con Carne

**Quick and Easy—Prepare Ahead**
**\* Beans, if tolerated**
**Makes 3 servings**
**\*\*Onion**

1/4 lb. LEAN GROUND BEEF
1 CLOVE GARLIC, minced
1/2 cup canned TOMATOES AND GREEN CHILES
1/2 cup ONION\*\*, chopped
1 can (16. oz.) KIDNEY\* BEANS IN TOMATO SAUCE (no
    added salt)
generous dash GROUND CUMIN

Combine beef with onion, garlic and cumin and cook at medium heat in a medium saucepan until beef is browned. Stir to break up meat. Then add remaining ingredients; bring to a boil and reduce heat. Simmer, uncovered, for 10 minutes, stirring occasionally to blend flavors.

SERVING SIZE: 1 cup

CALORIES: 232   CHOL.: 28 mg. FAT: 5.2 g. SODIUM: 72 mg.

# Beef Sandwich on Onion Bun

**Quick and Easy**
**Makes 1 serving**
**\*\*Onion bun**

*Preparing your own beef certainly lowers the percent of fat you find in  most fast foods.*

1 ONION BUN\*\*
2 oz. sliced LEAN BEEF
1 tsp. MUSTARD
2 TOMATO slices
1 GREEN PEPPER, sliced thin

Spread mustard on bun. Pile beef and tomato on bun. Top with green pepper. Try this sandwich with *Glazed Carrots* (see *Side Dishes*) and refreshing *Smorgasbord Cheese Cake* (see *Desserts*).

SERVING SIZE: 1 sandwich

CALORIES: 374   CHOL.: 35 mg. FAT: 8 g.  SODIUM: 183 mg.

\* = Dangerous to Some   \*\* = Consume with Caution   (see Pages 22 & 23)

# Citus Chops

Quick and Easy—Prepare Ahead
*Pork

**Makes 4 servings**    **Onion, orange peel, orange juice

*Because of changes in the pork industry, pork is no longer required to be cooked so long. Variation: substitute turkey ham for the pork.*

1/4 cup sliced GREEN ONION**
1 Tbsp. ORANGE PEEL**, grated
1 tsp. OIL
1/2 cup ORANGE JUICE**
4 lean, trimmed PORK LOIN CHOPS*
1/4 tsp. DRIED BASIL

Heat oil in large skillet. Add green onion and orange peel, sauté 3 to 4 minutes or until onion is almost tender. Remove onion and orange peel; set aside. Add pork chops and brown on both sides over medium heat; add onion and orange peel. Add orange juice and basil; cover and simmer for 10 minutes.

MICROWAVE: Omit oil; combine ingredients other than chops in a small bowl. Arrange chops in glass or ceramic dish with meaty parts to outside. Pour juice mixture over chops; cover with plastic wrap; poke holes in plastic wrap. Microwave on MEDIUM (50% power) for 8 to 10 minutes. Turn dish or rearrange chops. Replace plastic wrap and microwave for another 8 to 10 minutes.

Complete the meal with *Austrian Cooked Cabbage* (see *Side Dishes*) and *Mock Rice Pudding* (see *Desserts*).

SERVING SIZE: 1 pork chop

CALORIES: 222   CHOL.: 73 mg.  FAT: 12 g. SODIUM: 44 mg.

* = Dangerous to Some   ** = Consume with Caution   (see Pages 22 & 23)

# Favorite "Ham" Loaf

Specialty—Prepare Ahead
Makes 6 to 8 servings

*An old-time recipe, moist and tasty, that slices well.*

1 lb. ground SMOKED TURKEY
HAM
1/2 lb. TURKEY SAUSAGE
1/2 lb. GROUND BEEF
1/4 cup chopped PIMENTO
3/4 cup BREAD CRUMBS
3/4 cup MILK

1/2 tsp. SALT
1/4 chopped GREEN
PEPPER
1 EGG
2 Tbsp. MUSTARD
1/4 cup CATSUP

**Glaze:** 1 cup drained, crushed pineapple mixed with 1/3 cup brown sugar.

Combine ingredients and press into a large 8-1/2 inch x 4-1/2 inch loaf pan. Bake 1 hour at 350 degrees or until loaf pulls away from edges. Ten minutes before the loaf is done, glaze with brown sugar topping. If desired; baste 2 or 3 times.

SERVING SIZE: 1 slice

CALORIES: 247 (approx.)　　CHOL.: 92 mg.　　FAT: 14 g.
SODIUM: 326 mg.

# Pork Stir-Fry

Quick and Easy
Makes 4 servings　　　　　　　　　　　　　　　　*Pork

1 lb. trimmed, boneless PORK TENDERLOIN*, cut
crosswise into 1/4-inch strips
1 Tbsp. VEGETABLE OIL
1 pkg. (16 oz.) frozen STIR-FRY VEGETABLES or 3 cups
FRESH VEGETABLES cut into small pieces
SALT to taste

Heat oil over high heat in wok or large skillet. Quickly brown pork strips, stirring constantly. Add vegetables (thawed); cover and steam for 3 to 5 minutes or until vegetables are heated through but still crisp-tender. Fresh vegetables will take longer to cook. Add salt, cook and stir one minute.

SERVING SIZE: 6 ounces

CALORIES: 186　CHOL.: 74 mg.　FAT: 7 g.　SODIUM: 95 mg.

* = Dangerous to Some　　** = Consume with Caution　　(see Pages 22 & 23)

# Flank Steak with Mushrooms

**Makes 4 servings**

*Broiling meat is one of the most successful ways to cut down on fat. Not only is the meat not cooked in fat, but the excess fat drips through the broiler rack.*

**2 Tbsp. MARGARINE**
**1/4 cup chopped ONION****
**1/3 cup APPLE JUICE**
**1 lb. fresh MUSHROOMS*, sliced**
**1 lb. FLANK STEAK**
**PARSLEY SPRIGS**

Melt 2 tablespoons margarine in a large skillet over medium heat. Add mushrooms and onion; sauté, stirring occasionally, until tender and most of the mushroom liquid evaporates. Stir in apple juice and keep warm over low heat.

Broil steak 8 to 10 minutes on each side or to desired doneness. Cut into thin slices at an angle across grain. Serve topped with mushroom mixture and garnish with parsley sprigs.

SERVING SIZE: 4 ounces

CALORIES: 268   CHOL.: 58 mg.   FAT: 16 g.   SODIUM: 99 mg.

* = Dangerous to Some   ** = Consume with Caution   (see Pages 22 & 23)

# Mexican Beef Stir-Fry

**Quick and Easy**

**Makes 4 servings**                                              **\*\*Onion**

*Fork-tender, full of flavor and nutritious; this colorful dish is served on a bed of lettuce.*

**1 lb. well-trimmed TOP ROUND BEEF STEAK**
**1 tsp. DRIED OREGANO LEAVES**
**1 RED BELL PEPPER, cut into thin strips**
**1 medium ONION\*\*, cut into thin wedges**
**1 Tbsp. VEGETABLE OIL**
**1 tsp. GROUND CUMIN**
**1/8 tsp. GARLIC POWDER**
**1 to 2 JALAPEÑO PEPPERS, cut into slivers**
**ROMAINE LETTUCE, cut 1/4-inch thick**

Cut round steak into 1/8-inch thick strips. Combine oil, cumin, oregano and garlic; reserve half. Heat half of the seasoned oil in large non-stick frying pan over medium-high heat until hot. Add red pepper, onion and jalapeno pepper; stir-fry 2 to 3 minutes or until crisp-tender. Remove vegetables and set aside.

In same pan, stir-fry beef strips (half at a time) in reserved seasoned oil for 1 to 2 minutes. Return vegetables to pan and heat through. Serve beef mixture on a bed of lettuce.

SERVING SIZE: 4 ounces

CALORIES: 232   CHOL.: 65 mg.  FAT: 12 g.   SODIUM: 34 mg.

---

\* = Dangerous to Some    \*\* = Consume with Caution    (see Pages 22 & 23)

# Pork Tenderloin with Orange Marmalade Sauce

Quick and Easy
*Pork

Makes 4 servings      **Orange, orange marmalade

*The popular kiwi fruit is even more laden with vitamin C than oranges.*

1 lb. PORK* TENDERLOIN, trimmed and cut into 8 pieces
6 Tbsp. ORANGE MARMALADE**
2 KIWI FRUIT, peeled, thinly sliced
ORANGE* segments (optional)
1 Tbsp. MARGARINE
1 Tbsp. CATSUP
2 Tbsp. WHITE VINEGAR
1/2 tsp. HORSERADISH
1/8 tsp. GARLIC POWDER
CAYENNE PEPPER, to taste

Press each pork tenderloin slice to 1-inch thickness. Lightly sprinkle both sides of each slice with cayenne pepper. Heat margarine in large heavy skillet over medium-high heat. Add pork slices; cook 3 to 4 minutes on each side.

Combine orange marmalade, vinegar, catsup, horseradish and garlic powder in small saucepan. Simmer over low heat about 5 minutes, stirring occasionally. Place cooked pork slices on warm serving plate; spoon sauce over; top each slice with a kiwi slice. Garnish with remaining kiwi slices and orange segments, if desired.

MICROWAVE: Prepare pork slices as above. Melt margarine in large microwave-proof dish; add pork slices, cover and cook 6 to 8 minutes on HIGH (100% power). Turn dish and meat every 3 minutes. Combine marmalade, vinegar, catsup, horseradish and garlic powder in small bowl. Microwave 1 to 2 minutes, stirring occasionally. Place pork slices on warm serving platter and garnish and serve as above.

SERVING SIZE: 4 ounces

CALORIES: 267   CHOL.: 74 mg.  FAT: 7 g.  SODIUM: 136 mg.

* = Dangerous to Some   ** = Consume with Caution   (see Pages 22 & 23)

# Savory Beef Burgers

**Makes 4 servings**

Quick and Easy
**Onion

*Mama mia! What a burger! And, of course, have at hand the catsup, etc. for burger purists.*

1 lb. EXTRA LEAN GROUND BEEF
2 Tbsp. INSTANT MINCED ONION**
1 Tbsp. DIJON MUSTARD
4 TOMATO slices, 1/4-inch thick
1/4 tsp. GROUND CUMIN
1/4 tsp. CRACKED BLACK PEPPER
4-8 LETTUCE LEAVES
3/4 tsp. DRIED ITALIAN SEASONING
4 thin RED ONION RINGS**
4 BURGER BUNS

Combine ground beef, onion, mustard, Italian seasoning, cumin, pepper and salt. Mix lightly but thoroughly. Divide beef mixture into 4 equal portions and form into patties. Place patties on rack in broiler pan so surface of meat is 3 to 4 inches from heat. Broil 8 to 10 minutes, turning once.

Assemble burger submarine sandwich style. Serve immediately.

MICROWAVE: Prepare ground beef mixture as above. Place patties in a microwave-safe baking dish. Cook on HIGH (100% power) 8 minutes, turning dish after first 4 minutes. Assemble and serve as above.

SERVING SIZE: 1 burger

CALORIES: 239   CHOL.: 81 mg.  FAT: 13 g.  SODIUM: 90 mg.

---

* = Dangerous to Some   ** = Consume with Caution   (see Pages 22 & 23)

# Savory Brushed Steak

**Makes 8 servings**                    **\*\*Onion, lemon juice**

*Flank steak is another lean steak; flank steak may be a tough or tender steak depending on how the animal was exercised, age, type, etc. Note the market's tenderness category.*

1/4 cup MARGARINE
1/4 cup minced ONION\*\*
1/4 tsp. MARJORAM LEAVES
1/4 tsp. GROUND BLACK PEPPER
1 (2 lb.) FLANK STEAK, 1-1/2 to 2 inches thick
1/4 cup LEMON JUICE\*\*
1/2 tsp. OREGANO LEAVES
1/4 tsp. THYME LEAVES
1 small CLOVE GARLIC, minced

Melt margarine and mix in onion, lemon juice, oregano, marjoram, thyme, pepper and garlic. Transfer sauce to a heavy plastic bag. Place steak in bag and seal closed. Turn bag to coat meat evenly with marinade. Let stand at room temperature thirty minutes.

Remove meat from bag; place on broiling rack. Remove excess marinade from bag. Brush surface of meat with half the marinade. Broil for 7 minutes; turn and brush with remaining marinade. Broil about 7 to 8 minutes longer or to desired doneness.

SERVING SIZE: 4 ounces

CALORIES: 256    CHOL.: 58 mg.  FAT: 18 g. SODIUM: 118 mg.

* = Dangerous to Some    \*\* = Consume with Caution    (see Pages 22 & 23)

# Spicy Pot Roast with Dumplings

Specialty
*Curry powder
**Onion

**Makes 12 servings**

*A dish to prepare when you have the energy and the time.*

**Pot Roast:**
- 2 Tbsp. MARGARINE
- 3 lbs. POT ROAST OF BEEF
- 1 (16 oz.) can LOW-SODIUM TOMATOES, undrained
- 2 cups sliced ONIONS**
- 2 tsp. CURRY POWDER*
- 1 tsp. SUGAR

**Dumplings:**
- 1-1/2 cups ALL-PURPOSE FLOUR
- 1 Tbsp. LOW-SODIUM BAKING POWDER
- 1 Tbsp. MARGARINE
- 1 cup SKIM MILK
- 2 Tbsp. finely chopped ONION**
- 2 Tbsp. chopped PARSLEY
- 2 Tbsp. PIMENTO pieces
- 1 cup HOT WATER

In large heavy pan, melt 2 tablespoons margarine over medium high heat. Add beef and brown on all sides. Add tomatoes and sliced onions; bring to a boil. Reduce heat, cover and simmer for 2 hours. Stir in curry powder and sugar. Cover and cook an additional 1/2 hour. Place roast on serving platter and keep warm.

Dumplings: Combine flour and baking powder in a small bowl. Cut in margarine using a pastry blender or 2 knives. Stir in milk, chopped onion, parsley and pimento pieces until moistened.

Add hot water to gravy mixture in pot; bring to a boil. Drop batter by tablespoonfuls into boiling gravy in pot. Cover, cook over low heat for 15 minutes. Arrange dumplings around pot roast on platter. Slice roast and serve with tomato gravy.

SERVING SIZE: 1 cup

CALORIES: 267    CHOL.: 69 mg.    FAT 9 g.    SODIUM: 117 mg.

* = Dangerous to Some    ** = Consume with Caution    (see Pages 22 & 23)

# Tacos

**Makes 6 servings**

*A Mexican specialty, so popular and tasty that it's had a restaurant chain named for it.. To lower calorie count, use soft taco shells that haven't been fried.*

1 lb. EXTRA-LEAN GROUND BEEF
2 CLOVES GARLIC, minced
2 tsp. DRIED LEAF OREGANO
6 drops HOT PEPPER SAUCE
1/2 cup TOMATO SAUCE
1/2 cup chopped TOMATOES
1 medium ONION**, chopped
2 tsp. CHILI POWDER
1/2 tsp. GROUND CUMIN
1/4 tsp. SALT
6 TACO SHELLS
1 cup shredded LETTUCE
6 Tbsp. LOW-FAT COTTAGE CHEESE

Cook crumbled ground beef in a large skillet at medium heat, until it begins to lose its pink color. Add onion and garlic. Cook until onion is translucent. Drain fat off. Add chili powder, oregano, salt, hot pepper sauce, cumin and tomato sauce and simmer about 10 minutes.

Fill each taco shell with 1/3 cup of cooked mixture. Top with shredded lettuce, chopped tomato and 1 tablespoon cottage cheese.

SERVING SIZE: 1 taco

CALORIES: 230   CHOL.: 60 mg.  FAT: 9 g.  SODIUM: 210 mg.

* = Dangerous to Some   ** = Consume with Caution   (see Pages 22 & 23)

# Texas Meatloaf

**Makes 8 servings**

*Here's a recipe the whole family will enjoy. You can bake it in four small individual loaves or double the recipe to have an extra loaf for the freezer.*

1 1/2 lbs. LEAN GROUND BEEF
2 Tbsp. CORN OIL
1 GREEN PEPPER, coarsely chopped
1 large chopped ONION**
3 CLOVES GARLIC, minced or pressed
1 can (4 oz.) chopped GREEN CHILES, undrained
NON-STICK OIL COOKING SPRAY
3/4 cup OLD-FASHIONED OATS
3/4 cup BARBECUE SAUCE, divided
2 EGG WHITES (or 2 EGGS, or 1/4 cup EGG SUBSTITUTE)

Spray 8-1/2 x 4-1/2 x 2-1/2 inch loaf pan with cooking spray. In large skillet heat corn oil over medium heat. Add pepper, onion and garlic. Sauté 4 to 5 minutes or until tender. Remove from heat. In large bowl combine ground beef, egg whites, oats, 1/2 cup barbecue sauce and chiles. Stir in cooked vegetables. Spoon into loaf pan. Bake at 350 degrees oven 1 hour. Drain off excess liquid. Invert loaf onto serving platter. Spoon remaining 1/4 cup barbecue sauce over loaf. Let stand 10 minutes before slicing. Serve with *Lemon-Herb Twice-Baked Potato* (see *Side Dishes*).

SERVING SIZE: 4 ounces

CALORIES: 260   CHOL.: 55 mg.  FAT: 12 g. SODIUM: 410 mg.

---

* = Dangerous to Some   ** = Consume with Caution   (see Pages 22 & 23)

# Veal Scallopini

**Makes 4 servings**

*If veal is difficult to find in your market, substitute cube steak. The beef flavor is a little more "hearty", but both veal and cube steak are lower in fat content than most beef cuts.*

**1/2 lb. fresh MUSHROOMS*, sliced**
**1/4 cup ALL-PURPOSE FLOUR**
**1/8 tsp. GROUND BLACK PEPPER**
**1 Tbsp. WATER**
**3 Tbsp. MARGARINE**
**1 lb. thinly sliced VEAL CUTLETS**
**1/4 cup WHITE VINEGAR**
**Chopped PARSLEY**

Melt 1 tablespoon margarine in a large skillet over medium heat. Add mushrooms and sauté until tender; remove from pan.

Combine flour and pepper; coat veal with flour mixture. Melt remaining margarine in non-stick skillet and brown veal, a few pieces at a time, until done; remove from pan. Add vinegar and water to skillet, stirring until liquid is slightly thickened. Return veal and mushrooms to pan to heat through. Arrange on a serving platter and garnish with chopped parsley.

SERVING SIZE: 4 ounces

CALORIES: 302   CHOL.: 81 mg.   FAT: 18 g. SODIUM: 153 mg.

* = Dangerous to Some   ** = Consume with Caution   (see Pages 22 & 23)

# Poultry Entrées

# Barbecued Chicken

**Easy**
**Prepare Ahead**
**Makes 8 servings**                                    **\*\*Onion**

*A chicken dish that tastes good hot or cold. May also be frozen and reheated later.*

1/4 cup chopped ONION\*\*
1/2 cup LOW-SODIUM TOMATO JUICE
1/2 cup (4 cubes) frozen *LOW-SODIUM TOMATO BASE*
  (see *Sauces, Toppings*) or BARBECUE SAUCE
1/4 tsp. DRY MUSTARD
1/8 tsp. GARLIC POWDER
2 Tbsp. MARGARINE
2 Tbsp. diced GREEN PEPPER
2 Tbsp. firmly packed DARK BROWN SUGAR
2 Tbsp. WHITE VINEGAR
1 3-lb. CHICKEN, cut up
1/8 tsp. GROUND BLACK PEPPER

In small saucepan, melt margarine over medium heat. Add onion and green pepper; sauté until tender. Stir in tomato juice, tomato base, brown sugar, vinegar, dry mustard, garlic powder and pepper. Reduce heat to low and simmer, stirring occasionally, until very thick, about 30 minutes. Place in blender or food processor container; process until very smooth.

Remove all visible fat and loose skin from chicken pieces. Arrange chicken on broiler pan and brush with prepared sauce. Broil 5 to 6 inches from heat source for 20 to 25 minutes. Turn pieces, brush again with remaining sauce and broil for 20 to 25 minutes more or until done. Serve hot or cold. Add *Apple-Glazed Acorn Squash* (see *Side Dishes*) and *Whole Grain Muffins* (see *Breads*) to round out this meal.

SERVING SIZE: 1/3 - 1/2 pound per person

CALORIES: 180   CHOL.: 66 mg. FAT: 4 g.  SODIUM: 105 mg.

\* = Dangerous to Some   \*\* = Consume with Caution   (see Pages 22 & 23)

# Broiled Chicken Mexicana

**Easy**
**Prepare Ahead**
**\*\*Green onions**

**Makes 4 servings**

*Plain, white chicken breasts can become boring; here is another way to prepare white-meat poultry.*

**2 whole boneless, skinless CHICKEN BREASTS (about 1 lb.)**
**1/4 cup chopped CILANTRO or PARSLEY**
**2  CLOVES GARLIC, minced or pressed**
**2 Tbsp. chopped, pickled JALAPEÑO PEPPERS**
**1/4 cup LIME JUICE\*\***
**1/4 cup VEGETABLE OIL**
**1/4 tsp. SALT**
**1/2 cup sliced GREEN ONIONS\*\***
**2 cups chopped TOMATOES**

Place chicken breasts in shallow baking dish. In small bowl combine lime juice, vegetable oil, cilantro, garlic, peppers and salt. Pour half over chicken. Cover and marinate at room temperature 30 minutes.

Meanwhile, prepare salsa by adding tomatoes and green onions to mixture remaining in bowl. Set aside. Remove chicken from marinade, reserving 2 tablespoons for basting. Discard remaining marinade. Broil or grill chicken 6 inches from heat, basting occasionally, 15 to 20 minutes or until done. Serve with salsa. Delicious with **Mexican Corn** (see *Side Dishes*) and **Cashew Raisin Nuggets** (see *Desserts*).

SERVING SIZE:  1/3 - 1/2 pound per person

CALORIES: 220   CHOL.: 65 mg.  FAT: 10 g. SODIUM: 330 mg.

\* = Dangerous to Some    \*\* = Consume with Caution   (see Pages 22 & 23)

# Chicken a la Divan

**Quick and Easy——Prepare Ahead**
**Makes 6 servings**

*Tasting very French, delicate but rich in flavor, this dish is still low in calories, cholesterol and fat.*

3 cups cooked fresh BROCCOLI SPEARS, or 2 (10 oz.) pkgs.
   frozen BROCCOLI SPEARS, cooked and drained
1-1/2 lbs. sliced cooked CHICKEN BREAST
1-1/2 cups SKIM MILK
3 Tbsp. MARGARINE
3 Tbsp. ALL-PURPOSE FLOUR
2 Tbsp. WHITE VINEGAR
1/2 cup EGG SUBSTITUTE, or 2 EGGS
PAPRIKA

Arrange broccoli in the bottom of a 2-quart shallow baking dish or 6 individual baking dishes. Place chicken slices over broccoli. Cover with foil and bake at 350 degrees for 20 minutes or until hot.

Melt margarine in saucepan. Blend in flour; cook over low heat, stirring, until smooth and bubbly. Remove from heat and gradually stir in milk. Return to heat and bring to boil, stirring constantly. Gradually blend about 1/2 the hot mixture into egg substitute, then combine with remaining hot mixture. Stir in vinegar. Spoon sauce over chicken and broccoli; sprinkle lightly with paprika and serve.

MICROWAVE: In 2-quart microwave-proof shallow baking dish, arrange broccoli. Place chicken slices over broccoli; cover. Microwave on HIGH (100% power) for 5 to 7 minutes or until hot, rotating dish 1/4 turn after 3 minutes. Let stand, covered, while preparing sauce.

In 1-quart microwave-proof glass measure, microwave margarine and flour on HIGH for 2 minutes, stirring after 1 minute. Gradually stir in milk. Microwave on HIGH for 3-1/2 to 4-1/2 minutes, stirring every minute until thick and bubbly. Blend into egg substitute and proceed as above.

SERVING SIZE: 1 cup
CALORIES: 192   CHOL.: 49 mg.  FAT: 6 g.  SODIUM: 130 mg.

* = Dangerous to Some  ** = Consume with Caution  (see Pages 22 & 23)

# Chicken and Mushroom Dijon

**Makes 4 servings**

*This recipe will please your taste buds; yet is so quick and easy to prepare.*

2 Tbsp. MARGARINE
2 whole boneless skinless CHICKEN BREASTS, cut in
    half (about 1 lb.)
2 cups sliced fresh MUSHROOMS*
1 Tbsp. DIJON MUSTARD
1 small ONION**, chopped
1 tsp. CORNSTARCH
2/3 cup CHICKEN BROTH

In large skillet melt margarine over medium heat. Add chicken; sauté, turning frequently, 5 to 7 minutes or until done. Remove chicken. Add mushrooms and onion to skillet sauté 3 minutes.

In small bowl, stir chicken broth and cornstarch until smooth; whisk in mustard. Stir into mushroom mixture. Stirring constantly, bring to boil and boil 1 minute. Serve over chicken.

Add **Grilled Zucchini** (see *Side Dishes*) and **Strawberry-Banana Salad** (see *Salads*) to complete your meal.

SERVING SIZE: 1/2 chicken breast

CALORIES: 210  CHOL.: 65 mg.  FAT: 8 g.  SODIUM: 410 mg.

* = Dangerous to Some   ** = Consume with Caution   (see Pages 22 & 23)

# Chicken Breasts with Mushroom-Apple Juice Sauce

**Easy—Prepare Ahead**
**\*Mushrooms**
**Makes 4 servings**　　　　　　　　　　**\*\*Onion**

*A complete, tasty meal with a different flavor. The mushrooms add texture and the parsley contrast in color.*

**2 Tbsp. ALL-PURPOSE FLOUR**
**2 CHICKEN BREASTS, skinned, boned and split in half (about 1 lb. boneless)**
**2 cups thinly sliced MUSHROOMS\***
**2 cups hot COOKED RICE (prepared without added salt)**
**1/8 tsp. GROUND BLACK PEPPER**
**1/4 cup chopped ONION\*\***
**2 Tbsp. MARGARINE**
**1 cup APPLE JUICE**
**1/4 cup minced PARSLEY**

Combine flour and pepper; coat chicken breasts with mixture. Shake off and reserve excess flour.

Heat margarine in a large skillet over medium heat. Brown chicken on both sides, remove from skillet. Add mushrooms and onion to skillet. Sauté until tender and golden. Stir in reserved flour; blend in apple juice. Bring to a boil, stirring frequently. Return chicken to skillet with 2 tablespoons parsley. Cover; reduce heat and simmer for 25 minutes or until chicken is tender.

Serve over rice; garnish with remaining parsley.

SERVING SIZE: 1/2 chicken breast and 1/2 cup rice

CALORIES: 316　CHOL.: 66 mg. FAT: 7 g. SODIUM: 127 mg.

* = Dangerous to Some　\*\* = Consume with Caution　(see Pages 22 & 23)

# Chicken Cacciatore

**Makes 6 servings**

*The wonderful aroma of the onion, spices and chicken throughout the house will have everyone ready for this great Italian dish.*

**3 whole CHICKEN BREASTS, split and skinned
(about 3 lbs.)
1/2 cup diced GREEN PEPPER
1/2 tsp. OREGANO LEAVES
1/2 tsp. BASIL LEAVES
1/4 tsp. GROUND BLACK PEPPER
1/4 tsp. CELERY SEED
3 Tbsp. MARGARINE
1 cup sliced ONION**
1 CLOVE GARLIC, crushed
1 BAY LEAF
2 Tbsp. ALL-PURPOSE FLOUR
1 (16 oz.) can LOW-SODIUM TOMATOES, undrained
chopped PARSLEY**

Remove fat from chicken. Melt margarine in skillet; brown both sides of chicken. Remove.

Add onion, green pepper and garlic to skillet. Sauté until onion is tender. Stir in seasonings and tomatoes. Add chicken; bring to boil. Cover; reduce heat and simmer for 1 hour, turning chicken halfway through cooking. Remove bay leaf. Remove chicken to serving platter.

Blend together flour and small amount of sauce from skillet; stir into mixture in skillet. Cook until thickened, about 3 minutes. Pour over chicken; garnish with parsley.

Add a crusty bread and a tossed salad. Top off the meal with ***Cannoli Cream*** (see *Desserts*).

SERVING SIZE: 1 cup

CALORIES: 213    CHOL.: 66 mg.    FAT: 7 g.    SODIUM: 132 mg.

* = Dangerous to Some    ** = Consume with Caution    (see Pages 22 & 23)

# Chicken Egg Sandwich

**Quick and Easy**
**Makes 4 servings**

*This recipe makes a hearty, juicy sandwich.*

8 slices SALT-FREE WHOLE WHEAT BREAD
1/2 carton hard-cooked EGG SUBSTITUTE, or 2 EGGS,
    hard-cooked and sliced
1 medium TOMATO, sliced
3/4 lb. sliced cooked CHICKEN BREAST
3 Tbsp. MARGARINE
4 LETTUCE LEAVES
GROUND BLACK PEPPER

*To hard cook egg substitute;* pour into a heavy 8-inch skillet. Cover tightly. Cook over very low heat 10 minutes. Remove from heat. Allow to stand, covered, for 10 minutes.

Spread one side of bread slices with margarine. Layer lettuce leaves, eggs or egg substitute, chicken and tomato slices on 4 slices whole wheat bread. Sprinkle lightly with pepper. Top with remaining bread slices. Cut into quarters and serve.

SERVING SIZE: 1 sandwich

CALORIES: 397    CHOL.: 24 mg.  FAT: 14 g. SODIUM: 138 mg.

---

* = Dangerous to Some   ** = Consume with Caution  (see Pages 22 & 23)

# Chicken in Minced Parsley Sauce

Quick and Easy
Prepare Ahead
**Makes 6 servings**                                              **Onion

*Here's a delicious twist on those chicken breasts you've been eating. The multi-colored peppers are also a treat to the eye.*

1 ea. small **GREEN, RED** and **YELLOW PEPPERS**, sliced
    into 1/4-inch rings
6 boneless, skinless **CHICKEN BREASTS** (1-1/2 lbs. total)
2 cups (two 8 oz. cans) **TOMATO SAUCE**
1 Tbsp. **OLIVE OIL**
1/2 cup minced fresh **PARSLEY**
1/2 cup coarsely chopped **ONION****
1 medium **GARLIC CLOVE**, crushed
1/8 tsp. **SALT**

In 12-inch skillet, sauté pepper rings in oil until slightly tender. Remove; drain on paper towels. Brown chicken breasts in remaining oil in skillet. Keep warm.

In blender container, process tomato sauce, parsley, onion, garlic and salt until smooth. Pour over chicken in skillet. Heat to boiling; reduce heat; boil gently 5 minutes or until chicken is tender. Place chicken breasts on serving platter; arrange peppers on top. Serve with remaining sauce.

SERVING SIZE: 1 chicken breast

CALORIES: 180   CHOL.: 66 mg.  FAT: 4 g.  SODIUM: 459 mg.

# Chicken Pot Pie

**Specialty—Prepare Ahead**
**\*\*Onion**

**Makes 8 servings**

1/2 cup sliced ONION\*\*
1/8 tsp. GROUND BLACK PEPPER
1/2 cup chopped CELERY
1/4 cup SKIM MILK
1 medium POTATO, peeled and cubed
1 (10 oz.) pkg. frozen CUT GREEN BEANS
1 BROILER-FRYER CHICKEN, cut up (3-1/2 lbs.)
1 cup WATER
1/4 cup ALL-PURPOSE FLOUR
1/2 cup chopped WHITE ONION\*\*
2 medium CARROTS, cut in chunks
1/4 cup chopped PARSLEY
dash POULTRY SEASONING
*SINGLE CRUST FLAKY PASTRY* (see *Desserts, Sweets*)

Remove visible fat from chicken. In a large heavy pan, combine chicken, sliced onion, celery, pepper, poultry seasoning and water. Bring to a boil; reduce heat; cover and simmer for 30 minutes or until chicken is tender. Remove chicken from broth; discard skin and bones, cutting meat into 1/2-inch cubes. Chill chicken and broth, separately.

Discard fat from chilled broth and bring to a boil over medium high heat; add onions, potato and carrots. Reduce heat and cook until vegetables are tender-crisp.

Blend flour with skim milk. Add a little broth to the flour mixture; mix well. Quickly stir flour mixture into broth and vegetables. Bring to a boil over high heat, stirring constantly. Reduce heat to medium low; add green beans, parsley and cubed chicken; simmer for 2 minutes.

Pour chicken mixture into a 2-quart shallow baking dish. Prepare pastry. Roll out to fit top of dish and prick with fork. Arrange pastry over chicken mixture; flute edges, pressing crust firmly to edge of baking dish. Bake at 425 degrees for 20 to 25 minutes or until crust is golden brown.

SERVING SIZE: 1/8 of pot pie

CALORIES: 329   CHOL.: 63 mg.   FAT: 13 g.   SODIUM: 145 mg.

* = Dangerous to Some   ** = Consume with Caution   (see Pages 22 & 23)

# Chicken Scampi

**Makes 4 servings**

*"Wok" your way to health with this tasty, complete meal for dinner (but it also makes a great second-day lunch)!*

**2 whole CHICKEN BREASTS, boned, skinned and cut into bite-sized pieces**
**1 large ONION**, sliced**
**1 large GREEN PEPPER, seeded and cut into bite-sized pieces**
**1/2 tsp. SALT**
**8 oz. LINGUINE**
**4 tsp. OLIVE OIL**
**16 oz. frozen BROCCOLI, chopped into bite-sized pieces**
**1/2 LEMON**, juiced, or 1 Tbsp. bottled LEMON JUICE****
**1/2 tsp. PEPPER**
**PAPRIKA**

Heat olive oil in large frying pan or wok over medium-high heat. Add onion, green pepper and chicken; stir-fry about 5 minutes, or until meat changes color. Add broccoli and stir-fry for about 4 minutes, or until tender. Sprinkle with lemon juice, salt and pepper.

Cook linguine in large pot of boiling water for 9 minutes or until tender; drain. Place linguine in large serving dish; top with chicken-vegetable mixture; sprinkle with paprika.

SERVING SIZE: 1-1/2 cups

CALORIES: 485   CHOL.: 70 mg. FAT: 10 g. SODIUM: 30 mg.

---

* = Dangerous to Some   ** = Consume with Caution   (see Pages 22 & 23)

# Herb Roasted Turkey & Potatoes

**Easy**
**Specialty**
****Onion salt**

**Makes 6 servings**

*A hearty meat and potatoes dish.*

1-1/2 lbs. fresh boneless **TURKEY BREAST ROAST,**
   **skinned**
3/4 tsp. **DRIED OREGANO LEAVES**
4 **RED or WHITE POTATOES**
1/8 tsp. **GARLIC POWDER**
1/4 tsp. **ONION SALT****
2 Tbsp. **MARGARINE, melted**
**PAPRIKA**

Sprinkle garlic powder over surface of turkey. Place turkey in 9 x 9-inch pan; quarter potatoes and place around roast. Combine onion salt and oregano; sprinkle roast with 2/3 of the onion-oregano mixture. Drizzle margarine over potatoes and sprinkle with remaining onion-oregano mixture and paprika. Bake in 350 degree oven 1-1/2 hours or until it has an internal temperature of 170 degrees.

MICROWAVE: Prepare roast as above. Place in microwave-proof baking dish. Microwave on MEDIUM (50% power) for 18 to 20 minutes or until it has an internal temperature of 170 degrees. Turn dish every 5 to 6 minutes.

Complement this meal with *Festive Cranberry Sauce* (see *Sauces & Toppings*) and *Glazed Carrots* (see *Side Dishes*).

SERVING SIZE: 6 ounces

CALORIES: 280   CHOL.: 68 mg.  FAT: 12 g.  SODIUM: 69 mg.

* = Dangerous to Some  ** = Consume with Caution  (see Pages 22 & 23)

# Lemon Chicken

**Makes 4 servings**

*Lemon and chicken seem to have an affinity for each other.*

**1/2 cup LEMON JUICE****
**1/2 tsp. DRIED ROSEMARY**
**1 CHICKEN BROILER or FRYER cut in parts and skinned**
**1/8 tsp. GARLIC POWDER**
**1/2 tsp. DRIED PARSLEY**

Combine lemon juice, garlic, rosemary and parsley in a medium-sized glass or plastic dish. Arrange chicken parts in lemon mixture, turning to coat. Cover and refrigerate 10 to 20 minutes. Drain chicken, reserving lemon mixture. Broil or grill chicken 5 to 6 inches from heat, brushing with reserved lemon mixture. Continue cooking and basting until chicken is fork tender, about 35 to 45 minutes.

MICROWAVE: Prepare lemon mixture and chicken as above. After marinating chicken, place in microwave-safe dish, cover with vented plastic wrap; microwave on MEDIUM (50% power) for 16-20 minutes. Turn or rearrange chicken pieces so that less cooked parts are to the outside. Baste with reserved lemon mixture; replace wrap and continue cooking until chicken is fork tender, about 7 to 10 minutes more.

Peas seem to be a natural to serve with lemon chicken or try *Green Beans Delicious* (see *Side Dishes*).

SERVING SIZE: 1/4 chicken

CALORIES: 228   CHOL.: 102 mg.  FAT: 8 g. SODIUM: 77 mg.

* = Dangerous to Some   ** = Consume with Caution   (see Pages 22 & 23)

# Microwave Chicken Italiano

**Quick and Easy**
**Prepare Ahead**
**Makes 8 servings** **\*\*Onion**

*Another one-dish, low-calorie meal with zucchini, carrots and onion. Good as a leftover, too.*

8 CHICKEN BREAST HALVES, boned and skinned
  (2-1/2 to 3 lbs.)
1-1/4 cans (10-1/2 oz.) CHICKEN BROTH
1/8 tsp. PEPPER
2/3 cup (6 oz. can) TOMATO PASTE
1 medium ONION\*\*, sliced
1 cup (1 medium) ZUCCHINI, julienne
1-1/2 tsp. SEASONED SALT, divided
1/4 cup WATER
1/2 tsp. DRIED OREGANO LEAVES, crushed
1/2 tsp. DRIED BASIL
1 cup (2 medium) thinly sliced CARROTS
1 large GARLIC CLOVE, minced
pinch crushed RED PEPPER FLAKES (optional)

In 13 x 9 x 2-inch microwave-safe dish, place chicken breasts; season with 1 teaspoon seasoned salt and pepper. Distribute onion and carrot over chicken pieces; set aside.

In small bowl, blend tomato paste, chicken broth, water, remaining 1/2 teaspoon seasoned salt, oregano, basil, garlic and red pepper flakes, if desired. Pour over chicken, onion and carrots; cover, venting edge. Microwave on HIGH (100% power) for 10 minutes. Turn chicken pieces over and rearrange in dish. Cover and cook additional 7 minutes. Mix in zucchini; cover and cook 5 minutes or until chicken is cooked. Let stand, covered, 5 minutes before serving.

SERVING SIZE: 1 cup

CALORIES: 244   CHOL.: 107 mg.FAT: 3 g.   SODIUM: 777 mg.

# Orange Chicken Crepes

**Makes 4 servings**

Specialty
Prepare Ahead
**Onion, orange juice

*A festive dish for any meal—the seedless green grapes make a special effect and taste contrast.*

1-2/3 cups SKIM MILK
1-1/2 cups chopped cooked CHICKEN
1/4 cup ALL-PURPOSE FLOUR
3/4 cup SEEDLESS GREEN GRAPES, halved
2 Tbsp. minced PARSLEY
1/4 cup ORANGE JUICE**
1 Tbsp. MARGARINE
2 Tbsp. CHOPPED CELERY
2 Tbsp. chopped ONION**
8 PREPARED CREPES (see below)
dash GROUND BLACK PEPPER

Sauté celery and onion in margarine 2 to 3 minutes. Stir in flour and pepper. Gradually stir in milk. Bring to a boil, stirring constantly; cook 1 minute more. Remove from heat; stir in parsley.

Mix half the prepared sauce with chicken and grapes. Spoon chicken mixture on crepes; roll up and place in a greased 11 x 7 x 1-1/2 inch baking dish. Pour remaining sauce over crepes. Bake at 350 degrees for 20 minutes or until hot. Garnish with additional grapes, if desired.

## Crepes

Mix 2/3 cup skim milk, 2/3 cup all-purpose flour and 6 tablespoons egg substitute until smooth. Mix in 1 tablespoon melted margarine. Chill batter 30 minutes.

Melt 1/2 tablespoon margarine and lightly brush a heated 8 inch skillet. Pour in 2 tablespoons prepared batter; tip pan to spread mixture evenly. Cook until bottom is sightly browned. Turn and brown other side. Turn out onto waxed paper.

(Continued on next page)

* = Dangerous to Some   ** = Consume with Caution   (see Pages 22 & 23)

(Continued from previous page)

Repeat, brushing skillet with melted margarine as needed.

MICROWAVE: In 1-quart microwave-proof glass measure, place celery, onion, margarine, flour and pepper. Microwave on HIGH (100% power) for 1 minute. Gradually stir in milk. Microwave on HIGH for 6 to 8 minutes, stirring every 2 minutes until thick and bubbly. Stir in parsley. Prepare chicken mixture and fill crepes as above. Place crepes in greased 11 x 7 x 1-1/2 inch microwave-proof baking dish. Pour remaining sauce over crepes; cover, microwave on HIGH for 8 to 10 minutes, rotating 1/2 turn after 4 minutes. Let stand 5 minutes before serving.

SERVING SIZE: 2 crepes

CALORIES: 368   CHOL.: 50 mg. FAT: 11 g. SODIUM: 211 mg.

# Grilled Piquante Chicken

**Quick and Easy—Prepare Ahead**

**Makes 8 servings**

*For a taste bud treat try grilled poultry. Serve with julienne potatoes, zucchini and red pepper strips in foil packets.*

**4 CHICKEN BREASTS, skinned and boned and cut in half**
**2 packs SUGAR SUBSTITUTE**
**1 cup THICK SALSA**
**4 tsp. DIJON MUSTARD**

Mix salsa, sugar substitute and mustard. Marinate chicken breasts in this mixture for 2 hours in refrigerator.

When coals have turned white, place chicken breasts on barbecue grill. Turn after about 5 minutes. They should be done in 10 to 15 minutes.

Using a long-handled brush and wearing mitts, brush on marinade while grilling.

SERVING SIZE: 1/2 chicken breast

CALORIES: 154   CHOL.: 73 mg. FAT: 3 g.   SODIUM: 217 mg.

* = Dangerous to Some   ** = Consume with Caution   (see Pages 22 & 23)

# Oven-Crisp Chicken Breasts

**Quick and Easy—Prepare Ahead**
**Makes 8 servings**

*This recipe duplicates the flavor and crunch of deep-fat fried chicken without all the fat and calories.*

**1/2 cup SKIM MILK**
**2 EGG WHITES**
**1/2 cup ALL-PURPOSE FLOUR**
**1/2 tsp. SALT**
**1/4 tsp. PEPPER**
**8 boneless CHICKEN BREASTS (about 2 lbs.)**
**1 Tbsp. PAPRIKA**
**1 cup dry BREAD CRUMBS**
**1 tsp. DRIED BASIL LEAVES**
**1/4 cup VEGETABLE OIL**

Heat oven to 425 degrees. Rinse chicken breast halves; pat dry with paper towels.

Beat egg whites until frothy. Beat milk.

Combine flour, paprika, basil, salt and pepper in large plastic food storage bag. Place bread crumbs in another bag. Dip breast halves, one or two at a time, in flour mixture, then in egg white mixture, then in crumbs.

Place oil in 15-1/4 x 10-1/4 x 3/4 inch broiler pan or other shallow pan. Place in 425 degree oven for 3 or 4 minutes or until oil is hot, but not smoking. Add chicken breasts in single layer.

Bake at 425 degrees for 20 minutes; turn chicken over; bake for 5 minutes.

A perfect meal with a tossed salad, ***Lemon Garlic Asparagus*** (see *Side Dishes*) and ***Banana Cream Pie***(see *Desserts*).

SERVING SIZE: 1 chicken breast

CALORIES 240    CHOL.: 65 mg. FAT: 8 g.  SODIUM: 220 mg.

* = Dangerous to Some    ** = Consume with Caution    (see Pages 22 & 23)

# Poultry Sausage Patties

**Quick and Easy**
**Makes 8 servings**

*Try serving these poultry burgers like hamburgers.*

**3 Tbsp. MARGARINE**
**1 cup fresh BREAD CRUMBS**
**3 Tbsp. EGG SUBSTITUTE, or 1 large EGG**
**1 Tbsp. POULTRY SEASONING**
**2 tsp. GROUND SAGE**
**1/2 tsp. FENNEL SEED**
**1/4 tsp. GROUND BLACK PEPPER**
**1 lb. boneless uncooked CHICKEN BREAST, coarsely**
    **ground (or TURKEY)**
**1 tsp. BASIL LEAVES**

Melt 2 tablespoons margarine; combine with chicken and bread crumbs; set aside.

Crush spices together and mix with egg substitute; combine with chicken mixture; shape into 8 three-inch round patties, using about 2 tablespoons of mixture for each patty.

Melt remaining margarine in a large skillet over medium heat. Cook patties 5 to 8 minutes on each side, until lightly browned and cooked through. Serve hot.

MICROWAVE: Prepare patties as above. Omit remaining tablespoon margarine. Place 4 patties in 9-inch microwave-proof pie plate. Microwave on MEDIUM (50% power) for 8 to 12 minutes, rotating 1/2 turn after 1-1/2 minutes. Repeat with remaining patties.

Serve with ***Sweet Potatoes a la Orange*** (see *Side Dishes*) and ***Banana Snacking Cake*** (see *Desserts*).

SERVING SIZE: 1 patty

CALORIES: 121    CHOL.: 33 mg.  FAT: 5 g.  SODIUM: 111 mg.

* = Dangerous to Some   ** = Consume with Caution   (see Pages 22 & 23)

# Savory Lemon Chicken

Prepare Ahead
**Lemon juice

**Makes 4 servings**

*There never seems to be any of this dish left over. Have you ever noticed that it's the first one finished at a Chinese restaurant?*

**2 whole CHICKEN BREASTS, split and skinned (about 1-1/2 lbs.)**
**1 can (10-3/4 oz.) CREAM OF CHICKEN SOUP**
**1 Tbsp. chopped fresh PARSLEY**
**1/2 tsp. PAPRIKA**
**1 Tbsp. LEMON JUICE****
**1/4 cup chopped SWEET RED PEPPERS**
**4 LEMON SLICES** for garnish**
**VEGETABLE NON-STICK COOKING SPRAY**

Spray 10-inch skillet with vegetable cooking spray. Over medium heat, cook chicken 10 minutes or until browned on both sides.

In small bowl, combine soup, lemon juice and paprika. Stir into skillet. Reduce heat to low. Cover; simmer 25 minutes, stirring occasionally.

Add red pepper and parsley. Cover; cook 10 minutes or until chicken is fork-tender, stirring occasionally. Serve sauce over chicken. Garnish with lemon slices.

Add **Oriental Spinach** and **Parsley Potato Cakes** *(see Side Dishes)* to complement this dish.

SERVING SIZE:  1/2 chicken breast

**Recipe**
CALORIES:  221    CHOL.: 79 mg.  FAT: 8 g.  SODIUM:  417 mg.

**From Soup**
CALORIES:  72    CHOL.: 6 mg.  FAT: 5 g.  SODIUM:  351 mg.

* = Dangerous to Some    ** = Consume with Caution    (see Pages 22 & 23)

# Southwest Chicken

**Quick and Easy**
**Prepare Ahead**
**Makes 4 servings**

*An easy-to-prepare dish of tender chicken.*

**1-1/4 lbs. boneless CHICKEN BREASTS, skin removed**
**1 jar (12 oz.) CHUNKY SALSA (mild, medium, or hot)**
**VEGETABLE NON-STICK COOKING SPRAY**

Coat baking dish with non-stick vegetable spray. Place chicken in baking dish; spread salsa evenly over chicken. Marinate 1/2 hour, if possible. Preheat oven to 350 degrees. Bake 40 to 60 minutes.

MICROWAVE: Arrange chicken in microwave-safe baking dish; spread salsa evenly over chicken. Cover with waxed paper and refrigerate. Marinate 1/2 hour if possible. Remove from refrigerator and place in microwave. Cook on MEDIUM (50% power) for 10 minutes. Turn dish or rearrange chicken and cook for 8 minutes more or until tender.

*Jicama Salad* (see *Salads*) goes well here, with *Caramel Custard* (see *Desserts*) to top off the meal.

SERVING SIZE: 1 chicken breast

CALORIES: 199  CHOL.: 77 mg.  FAT: 4 g.  SODIUM: 265 mg.

* = Dangerous to Some   ** = Consume with Caution   (see Pages 22 & 23)

# Spicy Orange Turkey

**Quick and Easy**
**Prepare Ahead**
**Makes 4 servings**     **\*\*Onion powder, orange, orange juice, lemon juice**

*Another way of serving turkey so that it doesn't become boring. Your taste buds will be pleased by this variation.*

**12 oz. fully-cooked TURKEY BREAST, skinned**
**3 Tbsp. ORANGE JUICE CONCENTRATE\*\***
**1 tsp. CHILI POWDER**
**4 tsp. CORNSTARCH**
**1 large ORANGE\*\*, peeled and sliced crosswise**
**1/2 cup WATER**
**1/2 tsp. ONION POWDER\*\***
**1 Tbsp. LEMON JUICE\*\***
**1 medium GREEN PEPPER, cut into 1-inch chunks**

Cut turkey into 1/8-inch slices. Combine water, orange juice concentrate, lemon juice, chili powder, onion powder and cornstarch in skillet. Heat on medium, stirring constantly until thickened. Layer turkey, green pepper and orange slices in skillet. Bring to a boil; turn down heat. Cover; simmer 6 to 8 minutes. Place turkey in center of serving platter, place orange slices and green pepper around edge. Stir sauce, pour small amount over turkey. Place remaining sauce in bowl to be used over turkey as desired.

MICROWAVE: Cut turkey into 1/8-inch slices; combine water, orange juice concentrate, lemon juice, chili powder, onion powder and cornstarch in a microwave-safe baking dish. Cook 3 to 4 minutes on HIGH or until thickened. Stir every minute. Layer turkey, green pepper and orange slices in dish. Cook 6 to 8 minutes, turning dish every 2 minutes. Garnish and serve as above.

SERVING SIZE: 1/3 cup

CALORIES: 241    CHOL.: 68 mg.    FAT: 8 g.    SODIUM: 74 mg.

* = Dangerous to Some    ** = Consume with Caution    (see Pages 22 & 23)

# Stir-Fry Chicken and Broccoli

**Quick and Easy**
**Prepare Ahead**
****Green onions**

**Makes 4 servings**

*An Oriental way to prepare chicken; the combination of ingredients and aroma will have mouths watering throughout your home.*

1/4 tsp. GROUND GINGER
4 boneless, skinned whole CHICKEN BREASTS or 8
    THIGHS, skinned and boned
4 tsp. VEGETABLE OIL
1 cup CHICKEN BROTH, divided
1/4 tsp. PEPPER
1/2 tsp. SUGAR
16-20 oz. frozen BROCCOLI, bits and pieces
1 cup sliced GREEN ONION**
1 Tbsp. CORNSTARCH
SALT to taste

Cut chicken into bite-sized pieces; sprinkle with ginger and pepper. Heat oil in large frying pan or wok over high heat. Add chicken and stir-fry 3 minutes or until brown; remove from pan and set aside. Add broccoli and onion; stir-fry 3 minutes. Mix 3/4 cup chicken broth with salt and sugar. Stir in vegetables; return chicken to pan. Reduce heat to medium-high; cover and cook 2 minutes. Mix cornstarch and remaining 1/4 cup chicken broth. Stir into pan and cook, stirring for 1 minute. Remove from heat.

***Glazed Apple Tart*** (see *Desserts*) is a perfect finish for this meal.

SERVING SIZE: 1/2 cup broccoli and 1 chicken breast or 2 thighs.

CALORIES: 324   CHOL.: 97 mg.  FAT: 15 g. SODIUM: 286 mg.

* = Dangerous to Some  ** = Consume with Caution  (see Pages 22 & 23)

# Texas Style Duck

Specialty

**Makes 4-6 servings**                    **\*\*Onion, pecans, orange**

*A unique entrée specialty.*

## Stuffing:

1 cup diced CELERY
1 cup minced ONION\*\*
1-1/2 tsp. SALT
1/2 cup EGG SUBSTITUTE, or 2 EGGS
4 cups soft BREAD CRUMBS
1 cup coarsely chopped PECANS\*\*
1/2 cup MILK, scalded

Combine celery, onion, pecans, bread crumbs, salt; add to egg substitute. Mix well. Add scalded milk and blend.

SERVING SIZE: 1/2 cup

CALORIES: 160    CHOL. 0        FAT: 2 g.   SODIUM: 479 mg.

## Ducks

Two 2-1/2 lb. DUCKS
6 slices TURKEY BACON
1/2 cup CHILI SAUCE
1 cup CATSUP
ORANGE SLICES\*\*
PARSLEY

Stuff ducks—vent and neck—with stuffing. Sew up slits. Place 3 strips of bacon across the breast of each duck. Place on a rack in an uncovered roaster or baking pan. Roast in a very hot oven, 500 degrees, for 15 minutes. Then reduce to 350 degrees and roast until tender (allow 60 minutes per pound). A meat thermometer is helpful.

Remove bacon when it becomes brown. One-half hour before removing from oven, add catsup mixture and pour over

(Continued on next page)

---

\* = Dangerous to Some    \*\* = Consume with Caution    (see Pages 22 & 23)

(Continued from previous page)

duck.

Arrange duck on a hot platter; garnish with parsley and orange slices.

Serve with a watercress-grapefruit section salad with *Flavorful French Dressing* (see *Salads*), *Wild Rice Casserole* and *Green Beans Delicious* (see *Side Dishes*) and *Date-and-Nut Bread* (see *Breads*).

SERVING SIZE: 3-1/2 ounces

With skin
CALORIES: 337   CHOL.: 89 mg.  FAT: 28 g. SODIUM: 357 mg.

Without skin
CALORIES: 201   CHOL.: 84 mg.   FAT: 11 g. SODIUM: 60 mg.

# Turkey Quiche

**Easy—Prepare Ahead**
**Makes 6 servings**

*An excellent way to serve leftover turkey.*

**1 cup diced cooked TURKEY**
**1 cup SKIM MILK**
**1 carton (8 oz.) EGG SUBSTITUTE, or 4 EGGS**
**2 Tbsp. diced PIMENTOS**
**1/4 cup minced fresh PARSLEY**
**1/2 tsp. GROUND SAGE**
**1/8 tsp. GROUND BLACK PEPPER**
**1 9-inch *SINGLE CRUST FLAKY PIE CRUST* (see *Desserts*)**

Spread turkey in bottom of prebaked pie crust shell. Combine skim milk, egg substitute, parsley, pimento, sage and pepper; pour mixture over turkey. Bake at 350 degrees for 45 to 50 minutes or until knife inserted in center comes out clean. Allow to stand 10 minutes. Cut into wedges and serve.

SERVING SIZE: 1/6 of pie

CALORIES: 255   CHOL.: 18 mg.  FAT: 11 g. SODIUM: 178 mg.

* = Dangerous to Some   ** = Consume with Caution   (see Pages 22 & 23)

# Turkey Chili

**Makes 6 servings**

Quick and Easy
Prepare Ahead
*Kidney beans, if tolerated
**Onion

*Cooking time is less than one-half hour for this hearty, nutritious and popular dish.*

1/4 cup DRIED ONION**
1/4 tsp. GARLIC POWDER
1/2 medium GREEN PEPPER, chopped
1 can (6 oz.) TOMATO PASTE
1 can (15-1/2 or 16 oz.) KIDNEY* BEANS, with liquid
1/2 tsp. SALT
1/2 cup sliced CELERY
1 lb. GROUND TURKEY
1 can (12 oz.) TOMATO JUICE
1 tsp. GROUND CUMIN or CHILI POWDER
1 can (14-1/2 oz.) STEWED TOMATOES

Place ground turkey, onion, green pepper and celery in large skillet. Cook on medium heat for 10 minutes, stirring and separating turkey as it cooks. Add remaining ingredients. Bring to a boil, turn down heat. Simmer 5 minutes, stirring occasionally.

MICROWAVE: Place turkey, onion, green pepper and celery in large microwave-proof casserole. Cook for 6 minutes until no longer pink. Stir and separate turkey every 2 minutes. Add remaining ingredients; cover; cook 10 more minutes. Stir after 5 minutes.

Add *Baked Apple Crumble* or *Carrot Cake* (see *Desserts*) for a great finish to this excellent meal.

SERVING SIZE: 1-1/4 cups

CALORIES: 296   CHOL.: 47 mg.   FAT: 6 g.   SODIUM: 349 mg.

* = Dangerous to Some   ** = Consume with Caution   (see Pages 22 & 23)

# Turkey Steak Diane

**Makes 4 servings**

Quick and Easy
**\*\*Green onion**

*If you can't find fresh turkey breast steaks in the meat cuts, look for turkey (or chicken) tenders—the tenderloin muscle of poultry.*

2 Tbsp. MARGARINE, divided
3 Tbsp. chopped GREEN ONION\*\*
1 tsp. SALT
2 tsp. finely chopped PARSLEY, or 1/2 tsp. DRIED PARSLEY
1 lb. (4) fresh TURKEY BREAST STEAKS, skinned
2 Tbsp. WHITE VINEGAR
1 Tbsp. WATER

Melt 1 tablespoon margarine in skillet over medium heat. When margarine begins to bubble, add turkey; cook 3 minutes, turn. Turn down heat to medium-low; cover, cook 5 minutes more or until juices run clear. Melt remaining margarine in small saucepan; add green onion; cook over medium heat and stir 2 to 3 minutes. Add vinegar, water and salt; cook 2 minutes more. Serve over turkey steaks, sprinkle with parsley.

MICROWAVE: Melt 1 tablespoon margarine in microwave-safe dish on MEDIUM power; add turkey. Cover, cook 3 minutes, turn turkey over. Cook 3 more minutes. Let stand covered 5 minutes or until juices run clear. Melt remaining margarine in small microwave-safe dish on HIGH power. Add green onion; cook and stir 1 to 2 minutes. Add vinegar, salt and water and cook 1 to 2 minutes more. Serve over turkey steaks, sprinkle with parsley.

SERVING SIZE: 1 turkey steak

CALORIES: 199   CHOL.: 65 mg.  FAT: 9 g.  SODIUM: 130 mg.

# Fish Entrées

# Baked Halibut

**Quick and Easy**

**Makes 6 servings**               **\*\*Onion, lemon or lime juice**

*A delicious fish favorite, low in calories, salt and fat and still high in good taste.*

1/4 tsp. THYME, crushed
1/8 tsp. each ROSEMARY, SALT and PEPPER
2 medium ONIONS\*\*, thinly sliced or julienned
2 CARROTS, sliced or julienned
1 Tbsp. melted MARGARINE or BUTTER
2 to 2-1/2 lb. HALIBUT
2 stalks CELERY, sliced or julienned
2 Tbsp. LEMON or LIME JUICE\*\*

Combine thyme, rosemary, salt and pepper; season halibut with mixture. Place half of vegetables in baking dish; place halibut on vegetables. Top halibut with remaining vegetables; drizzle with lemon or lime juice and margarine. Bake at 450 degrees, allowing about 10 minutes cooking time per inch of thickness measured at its thickest part, or until halibut flakes easily when tested with a fork.

Serve with **Roasted Garlic Potatoes** (see *Side Dishes*), peas and **Lemon Love Notes** (see *Desserts*).

SERVING SIZE: 5 ounces

CALORIES: 254   CHOL.: 50 g.   FAT: 10 g. SODIUM: 222 mg.

\* = Dangerous to Some   \*\* = Consume with Caution   (see Pages 22 & 23)

# "Creamed" Tuna Over Toast

### Quick and Easy
### Makes 6 servings

*To save time, chicken soup may be substituted for the broth and flour. Toasted bread or muffins afford texture contrast with the creamed tuna and peas.*

**1-1/2 cups CHICKEN BROTH**
**1 can (6-1/2 oz.) WATER-PACKED TUNA, drained**
**3 Tbsp. FLOUR**
**2 cups FROZEN PEAS**
**6 slices BREAD or 6 MUFFIN halves**
**SEASONING to taste**

In saucepan, bring 1 cup of chicken broth to boil. In a bowl, combine the other 1/2 cup broth with 3 tablespoons flour. Mix until smooth. Add flour mixture to broth in saucepan; mix until smooth. Add tuna and peas, simmer 5 minutes. Adjust seasoning to taste. Toast the bread or English muffins; ladle creamed tuna mixture over toast or muffins.

SERVING SIZE: 2/3 cup sauce over base

CALORIES: 230    CHOL.: 13 mg.  FAT: 2 g.  SODIUM: 619 mg.

---

\* = Dangerous to Some    \*\* = Consume with Caution    (see Pages 22 & 23)

# Curried Shrimp and Rice

**Quick and Easy**
**Prepare Ahead**
**\*Vanilla extract, curry powder**

**Makes 8 servings**

*A one-dish meal that is a real winner (especially suitable for buffets) because it is equally good served with hot entrées or cold, as well as with salad.*

1 can (20 oz.) crushed PINEAPPLE, packed in juice, undrained
1/2 tsp. VANILLA EXTRACT*
1 can (6 oz.) WATER CHESTNUTS, drained and sliced
3 cups cooked BROWN RICE
2 tsp. CURRY POWDER*
1/2 tsp. SALT
1/2 tsp. COCONUT EXTRACT
3 cups (1 lb.) cooked SHRIMP

Preheat oven to 325 degrees. Combine pineapple and its juice with the curry powder, salt and extracts and mix well. Add water chestnuts, shrimp and rice and again mix well. Spoon into a casserole or baking dish and bake, uncovered, for 30 minutes.

SERVING SIZE: 1 cup

CALORIES: 191 CHOL.: 111 mg. FAT: 1 g. SODIUM: 278 mg.

* = Dangerous to Some  ** = Consume with Caution  (see Pages 22 & 23)

# Fillet of Sole Amandine

**Quick and Easy**

**Makes 4 servings**          **\*\*Almonds, scallions, lemon juice**

*The freshness of the fish is all important for taste. Also important is not overcooking fish. Cook only until it has lost its translucent color and is still moist and juicy.*

3 Tbsp. sliced ALMONDS\*\*
2 Tbsp. ALL-PURPOSE FLOUR
1 Tbsp. sliced SCALLIONS\*\*
1 lb. fresh SOLE FILLETS
1 Tbsp. MARGARINE
1 Tbsp. LEMON JUICE\*\*
dash GROUND BLACK PEPPER

In large skillet, toast almonds over low heat. Remove from skillet, set aside.

Cut fillets in half lengthwise. Combine flour and pepper; coat fillets with mixture. Melt margarine in skillet over medium heat. Sauté fillets until golden, turning once, about 2 to 3 minutes on each side. Remove from skillet to a warm platter.

Return almonds to skillet with scallions; toss and stir until warm. Spoon over fillets and sprinkle with lemon juice. Garnish with parsley and lemon wedges, if desired. Serve immediately.

SERVING SIZE: 4 oz.

CALORIES: 170   CHOL.: 54 mg.  FAT: 6 g.  SODIUM: 117 mg.

* = Dangerous to Some   \*\* = Consume with Caution   (see Pages 22 & 23)

# Fish Creole

**Makes 4 servings**

**Easy**
**\*\*Onion**

*These Neptune nibbles can be a healthy highlight of the week. Fish may not be a "brain food" but certainly is a smart choice.*

1 pkg. (16 oz.) frozen COD FILLETS
1-1/2 cups chopped ONIONS\*\*
4 medium ripe TOMATOES, peeled and coarsely chopped
2 tsp. PAPRIKA
1/8 tsp. GROUND RED PEPPER
1 Tbsp. CORNSTARCH
2 cups hot cooked RICE (prepared without added salt)
1 Tbsp. MARGARINE
2 CLOVES GARLIC, minced
1/2 cup chopped GREEN PEPPER
2 Tbsp. chopped PARSLEY
1/2 tsp. SUGAR
1 BAY LEAF
1 Tbsp. WATER

Partially thaw cod fillets, leaving in a block.

Melt margarine in a large saucepan; add onions, green pepper and garlic; sauté until tender, about 5 minutes. Add tomatoes, parsley, paprika, sugar, red pepper and bay leaf and bring to a boil. Reduce heat, cover, and simmer 30 minutes.

Cut partially thawed cod into 1-inch square pieces. Add to sauce; cook about 5 minutes, stirring occasionally, until fish flakes easily with a fork. Remove bay leaf. Blend together cornstarch and water; add to creole and cook, stirring until slightly thickened. Serve with rice.

MICROWAVE: in 2-quart microwave-proof casserole, melt margarine on HIGH (100% power) for 1/2 to 1 minute. Add onions, green pepper and garlic. Microwave on HIGH for 3-1/2 to 4-1/2 minutes until onion is translucent, stirring after 1-1/2 minutes. Add tomatoes, parsley, paprika, sugar, red pepper and bay leaf; cover. Microwave on HIGH for 10 to 12 minutes, stirring after 5 minutes.

(Continued on next page)

* = Dangerous to Some   \*\* = Consume with Caution   (see Pages 22 & 23)

(Continued from previous page)

Cut partially thawed cod into 1-inch square pieces. Add to sauce; cover. Microwave on HIGH for 1-1/2 to 2 minutes, stirring after 1 minute. Remove bay leaf; blend cornstarch and water; add to creole; cover. Microwave on HIGH for 1 minute or until slightly thickened. Let stand covered 3 to 5 minutes before serving.

SERVING SIZE: 1 cup

CALORIES: 293   CHOL.: 49 mg.   FAT: 4 g.   SODIUM: 98 mg.

# Fish 'n Veggie Bundles

Quick and Easy
*Mushrooms
Makes 4 servings                    **Green onion

*Seafood, the 1990's slim-down favorite, gives a feeling of "just-for-you" in these packets.*

4 FLOUNDER FILLETS (about 1 lb.)
1/4 lb. MUSHROOMS*, thinly sliced
1/2 cup chopped RED PEPPER
1/8 tsp. freshly ground PEPPER
4 tsp. MARGARINE
1/4 tsp. SALT
1/4 tsp. DRIED BASIL
1/4 cup sliced GREEN ONIONS**

Cut 4 (12-inch) lengths of aluminum foil. Place one fillet at short end of each piece of foil. Divide mushrooms, red pepper and green onions evenly over fillets. Sprinkle with basil, salt and pepper. Top each fillet with 1 teaspoon margarine. Bring other end of foil over and tightly seal to form a packet. Place packets on ungreased cookie sheet. Bake in 425 degree oven 10 to 12 minutes or until fish is firm but moist.

SERVING SIZE: 1 bundle

CALORIES: 150   CHOL.: 55 mg.   FAT: 5 g.   SODIUM: 260 mg.

* = Dangerous to Some   ** = Consume with Caution   (see Pages 22 & 23)

# Pasta Primavera with Salmon

Quick and Easy—Prepare Ahead
*Mushrooms
Makes 6 servings
**Onion, lime or lemon

*Protein, vegetables and starch for a complete meal.*

1-1/2 cups sliced MUSHROOMS*
1/2 cup frozen PEAS, thawed
1/2 cup diced TOMATO
1/8 tsp. BASIL, crushed
1 lb. SALMON, cooked and flaked or,
　　2 cans (6 oz.) WATER-PACKED TUNA, drained
1 small YELLOW SQUASH or ZUCCHINI, sliced and cooked
　　crisp-tender
2 tsp. instant minced or chopped ONION**
2 Tbsp. MARGARINE
1 Tbsp. FLOUR
1 tsp. PARSLEY FLAKES
1/2 cup 1% SKIM MILK
8 oz. SPINACH FETTUCCINE or SPAGHETTI, cooked
　　and drained
LIME or LEMON wedges** for garnish
SALT and PEPPER to taste

Sauté mushrooms and onion in margarine. Add flour, basil and oregano; cook and stir 1 minute. Gradually add milk; cook and stir until thickened. Add salmon, squash, peas, tomato and parsley. Heat thoroughly. Toss hot fettuccine with vegetable mixture. Season to taste with salt and pepper.

MICROWAVE: Melt margarine in medium microwave-proof bowl. Mix in mushrooms and onion; cook 2 to 3 minutes, stirring after 1 minute. Add flour, basil and oregano; cook for 30 seconds; stir. Gradually add milk; cook about 2 to 3 minutes or until thickened. Stir every minute. Add salmon, squash, peas, tomato and parsley; cook 4 to 5 minutes or until heated through. Toss hot fettuccine with vegetables; season to taste; garnish with lime or lemon wedges.

SERVING SIZE: 1-1/2 cups

CALORIES: 271　CHOL.: 68 mg. FAT: 8 g. SODIUM: 110 mg.

* = Dangerous to Some　** = Consume with Caution　(see Pages 22 & 23)

# Saucy Fish

Quick and Easy
*Mayonnaise (check label)
**Yogurt

**Makes 4 servings**

*An easy-to-prepare seafood dish that starts with frozen fillets!*

**1 lb. frozen COD FILLETS (non-breaded)**
**1 Tbsp. DIJON MUSTARD**
**1/2 cup PLAIN NONFAT YOGURT\*\***
**1 Tbsp. "light" or REDUCED-CALORIE MAYONNAISE\***
**Grated BLACK PEPPER**

Preheat oven to 350 degrees. Place fillets in baking dish. Mix remaining ingredients; pour mix over fillets. Bake for 25 to 35 minutes, or until fish flakes.

MICROWAVE: Arrange fillets in microwave-safe dish with thickest parts to the outside. Mix remaining ingredients; pour over fillets. Cover with vented plastic wrap. Microwave on HIGH (100% power) for 3 minutes. Turn dish or move less cooked parts to outside of dish. Re-cover and microwave 3 to 5 more minutes, or until fish flakes.

*Cajun Rice* (see *Vegetable Entrées*) and *Yellow Squash Fritters* (see *Side Dishes*) fit this recipe well. Especially when you add *Honey Walnut* or *Banana Snacking Cake* (see *Desserts*) for that final treat.

SERVING SIZE: 1/4 pound

CALORIES: 142   CHOL.: 63 mg.  FAT: 3 g.  SODIUM: 160 mg.

---

\* = Dangerous to Some   \*\* = Consume with Caution   (see Pages 22 & 23)

# Shrimp Sauté with Dijon Mustard

**Makes 4 servings**

Quick and Easy
**Lemon juice

*When shrimp are on sale, try this favorite. Your family will appreciate this universal favorite.*

**1 lb. large SHRIMP, peeled, deveined and butterflied**
**1/4 tsp. DRIED TARRAGON LEAVES**
**2 Tbsp. chopped PARSLEY or 1-1/2 tsp. DRIED PARSLEY**
**1 CLOVE GARLIC, crushed**
**2 Tbsp. MARGARINE**
**3 Tbsp. DIJON MUSTARD**
**1 Tbsp. LEMON JUICE****
**RICE, cooked**

In large skillet, heat margarine over medium-high heat. Add shrimp and garlic to margarine, sauté for 4 to 5 minutes or until shrimp are pink. Remove from heat; stir in mustard, parsley, lemon juice and tarragon. Serve immediately over rice.

MICROWAVE: In shallow 2-quart microwave-proof dish, microwave margarine on HIGH (100% power) for 30 seconds or until melted. Add shrimp and garlic; cover. Microwave on HIGH for 4 to 5 minutes or until shrimp are pink and tender. Stir in mustard, parsley, lemon juice and tarragon. Serve immediately over hot rice.

SERVING SIZE: 4 ounces

CALORIES: 143  CHOL.: 161 mg. FAT: 7 g.  SODIUM: 85 mg.

* = Dangerous to Some  ** = Consume with Caution  (see Pages 22 & 23)

# Sweet and Sour Fish

**Quick and Easy**
**\*Raisins**
**\*\*Onion**

**Makes 6 servings**

*Be sure the raisins, as well as all dried fruit, are soft and not hard and dried; sometimes fermentation has already begun. Rice is a good choice as an accompaniment.*

**1-1/2 cups WHITE VINEGAR**
**1/3 cup SUGAR**
**3/4 cup GOLDEN SEEDLESS RAISINS\***
**1-1/2 lb. WHITEFISH FILLETS**
**1/4 cup EGG SUBSTITUTE, or 1 EGG**
**3/4 cup WATER**
**2 cups sliced ONIONS\*\***
**2 Tbsp. MARGARINE**
**2 Tbsp. ALL-PURPOSE FLOUR**
**dash GROUND BLACK PEPPER**

In large saucepan, boil vinegar, water and sugar for 10 minutes. Add onions and raisins; cook 10 minutes. Add white-fish fillets; cover and simmer for 10 to 12 minutes. Remove fish; set aside. Strain out and set aside onions and raisins; reserve 1-1/2 cups liquid.

In small saucepan, melt margarine over medium heat. Stir in flour and pepper; cook 1 minute. Stir in reserved liquid and egg substitute. Cook and stir until thickened, about 2 to 3 minutes.

Pour sauce over fish; garnish with onions and raisins. Serve hot or at room temperature.

SERVING SIZE: 1-1/2 cups

CALORIES: 322   CHOL.: 68 mg.  FAT: 11 g. SODIUM: 107 mg.

* = Dangerous to Some   ** = Consume with Caution   (see Pages 22 & 23)

# Tuna Noodle Supreme

**Makes 6 servings**

*A one-dish seafood entrée, whose flavors blend well—peas, tuna and noodles. If desired, substitute mushroom soup for the cornstarch and milk (does increase sodium content).*

1 Tbsp. MARGARINE
2 cups sliced MUSHROOMS*
1 large RED PEPPER, diced
1 medium ONION**, chopped
2 cans (6-1/2 oz. each) WATER-PACKED TUNA, drained
    and flaked
8 oz. medium EGG NOODLES, cooked and drained
2 Tbsp. LEMON JUICE**
2 cups LOW-FAT MILK
2 Tbsp. CORNSTARCH
1 cup frozen PEAS, thawed
1/2 tsp. HOT PEPPER SAUCE

In medium skillet melt margarine over medium-high heat. Add mushrooms, red pepper and onion; sauté 4 to 5 minutes or until vegetables are tender. In small bowl combine milk, cornstarch and hot pepper sauce until smooth. Stir into vegetable mixture. Stirring constantly, bring to a boil and boil 1 minute. Reduce heat to low. Add tuna and peas; heat through. Stir in lemon juice. Serve over noodles.

SERVING SIZE: 1-1/4 cups sauce and noodles

CALORIES: 310   CHOL.: 50 mg.  FAT: 5 g.  SODIUM: 270 mg.

* = Dangerous to Some   ** = Consume with Caution   (see Pages 22 & 23)

# Whitefish Stew

**Quick and Easy**

Makes 7 servings

**\*\*Onion**

*Even cafeterias are now offering a fish stew—serve in bowls over fluffy rice for a flavorful, completely balanced meal.*

1-1/2 lbs. COD, POLLOCK, ROCKFISH FILLETS, defrosted and drained
2 medium GREEN PEPPERS, chopped
2 CARROTS, thinly sliced
1 can (28 oz.) TOMATOES
1 tsp. SUGAR
1 tsp. BASIL, crushed
1/2 cup WHITE VINEGAR or FISH STOCK
2 Tbsp. VEGETABLE OIL
1 large ONION\*\*, chopped
1 large CLOVE GARLIC, minced
1 can (12 oz.) TOMATO JUICE

Cut fish into 1-inch chunks. Heat oil in large pot; sauté green peppers, carrots, onion and garlic in oil until onion is tender. Add tomatoes, tomato juice, sugar and basil. Bring to boil; simmer 10 minutes. Add vinegar and fish; simmer 8 minutes longer, or until fish flakes easily when tested with a fork.

MICROWAVE: Prepare fish as above; mix with remaining ingredients except oil. Place in microwave-proof baking dish; cover with plastic wrap. Microwave on HIGH (100% power) for 3 to 4 minutes. Let stand, covered 1 to 2 minutes. Stir, add vinegar, and cook for 3 to 5 minutes more or until fish flakes easily.

Finish your meal with *Lemon Love Notes* (See *Desserts, Sweets*).

SERVING SIZE: 1-1/4 cups

CALORIES: 179   CHOL.: 52 mg.   FAT: 6 g.   SODIUM: 342 mg.

---

\* = Dangerous to Some   \*\* = Consume with Caution   (see Pages 22 & 23)

# Side Dishes

# Apple-Glazed Acorn Squash

**Quick and Easy**
**Makes 4 servings**

*A delicious variation for acorn squash, low in calories, and high in vitamin A's precursor, beta-carotene.*

**1 medium ACORN SQUASH (about 1/1-2 lb.)**
**2 Tbsp. frozen APPLE JUICE CONCENTRATE, thawed**
   **and undiluted**
**1/8 tsp. GROUND GINGER**
**1/8 tsp. CINNAMON**

Pierce whole squash with a fork several times, and place on a paper towel in microwave oven. Microwave at HIGH 4 minutes.

Cut squash into 4 wedges; discard seeds and membrane. Place, cut sides up, in an 11 x 7 x 2-inch baking dish. Pierce flesh several times with a fork; set aside.

Combine juice, cinnamon and ginger, stir well, and brush over squash. Cover with heavy-duty plastic wrap; microwave at HIGH 6 to 8 minutes or until tender, rotating dish a half-turn after 3 minutes. Spoon remaining sauce over squash.

SERVING SIZE: 1/4 squash

CALORIES: 63    CHOL.: 0    FAT: 0.2 g.    SODIUM: 6 mg.

---

* = Dangerous to Some    ** = Consume with Caution    (see Pages 22 & 23)

# Austrian Cooked Cabbage

**Quick and Easy**
**Makes 2 servings**

*Cabbage is an inexpensive source of vitamin C and an anti-cancer, cruciferous vegetable.*

**3 cups shredded RED CABBAGE**
**1 tsp. CLOVES**
**1/4 cup WHITE VINEGAR**
**1 tart APPLE, chopped**
**VEGETABLE COOKING SPRAY**

Sauté cabbage until tender in a non-stick pan sprayed with vegetable cooking spray. Add vinegar, apple and cloves. Simmer until desired texture.

SERVING SIZE: 1 cup

CALORIES: 90    CHOL. 0    FAT: 1 g.    SODIUM: 38 mg.


# Baby Carrots with Dill

**Quick and Easy**
**Makes 4 servings**

*A simple way to make carrots "gourmet". Chefs define "gourmet" as interesting (not necessarily expensive, difficult to prepare, or foreign!)*

**1 lb. BABY CARROTS**
**2 Tbsp. FRESH DILL, chopped, or 1/2 tsp. DRIED DILL**
**WATER**

Steam scrubbed (but not peeled) baby carrots and dill in steamer or covered saucepan (use 1 inch water) until tender. Serve hot or cold.

SERVING SIZE: 2/3 cup

CALORIES: 42    CHOL.: 0    FAT: 0    SODIUM: 47 mg.

* = Dangerous to Some    ** = Consume with Caution    (see Pages 22 & 23)

# Cinnamon Apples

**Makes 2 servings**

**Quick and Easy**
**\*\*Lemon juice**

*When an apple has lost its crispness, bake it, or make this welcome addition to any meal, hot or cold.*

1 medium unpeeled tart APPLE, thinly sliced
1/8 tsp. GROUND CINNAMON
2 tsp. LEMON JUICE\*\*
1 tsp. MARGARINE
2 Tbsp. SUGAR (or sweetener to taste)

Toss apple with lemon juice, set aside. Melt margarine in a non-stick skillet over medium heat. Add sugar and cinnamon; stir well. Add apple, cook 7 minutes or until tender, stirring occasionally.

SERVING SIZE: 1/3 cup

CALORIES: 106    CHOL.: 0    FAT: 2.1 g.    SODIUM: 23 mg.


# Grilled Zucchini

**Makes 6 servings**

**Easy**
**\*\*Lime juice**

*Another great way to serve zucchini.*

1 lb. ZUCCHINI, small
1 tsp. OREGANO, dried
2 Tbsp. OLIVE OIL
1 LIME\*\*, juiced
SALT and PEPPER to taste

Slice zucchini in half lengthwise. Rub with olive oil. Sprinkle with pepper; let rest for about 30 minutes.

Preheat broiler. Place zucchini on baking pan, cut sides up. Broil close to the heat until well browned. Remove from heat; sprinkle with lime juice. Season to taste.

SERVING SIZE: 1/2 cup

CALORIES: 58    CHOL.: 0    FAT: 4 g.    SODIUM: 2 mg.


\* = Dangerous to Some    \*\* = Consume with Caution    (see Pages 22 & 23)

# Glazed Carrots

Quick and Easy
* Orange peel
**Walnuts

**Makes 6 servings**

*A beautiful, crunchy way to serve carrots. Remember that cornstarch or flour must be mixed with cold water (or fat) before adding to a hot mixture, and then brought to a boil to cook the starch.*

1 lb. CARROTS, scraped and thickly sliced (about 3-1/2 cups)
1/4 cup firmly packed LIGHT BROWN SUGAR
2 Tbsp. WALNUTS**, chopped
1 Tbsp. MARGARINE
1 Tbsp. grated ORANGE PEEL**
WATER

Cook carrots in small amount of unsalted water just until tender-crisp. Drain well.

Melt margarine in a large skillet; stir in brown sugar and orange peel; cook until sugar melts and mixture thickens. Add carrots and cook over low heat for 10 minutes, stirring occasionally, until tender and glazed. Top with walnuts and serve.

MICROWAVE: In 1-quart microwave-proof casserole, cover and microwave carrots, margarine and brown sugar on HIGH (100% power) for 9 to 11 minutes, stirring after 5 minutes.

Blend 2 tablespoons cold water and 1-1/2 teaspoons cornstarch until smooth; stir into carrot mixture with orange peel and walnuts; cover. Microwave on HIGH for 2 to 4 minutes or until thickened. Stir before serving.

SERVING SIZE: 2/3 cup

CALORIES: 97    CHOL.: 0    FAT: 8 g.    SODIUM: 42 mg.

* = Dangerous to Some   ** = Consume with Caution   (see Pages 22 & 23)

# Green Beans Delicious

**Makes 6 servings**

*This recipe is really a winner; frozen green beans are also successful. For guests, prepare the sautéed vegetables the day before and cook the beans on the day of the party.*

1 lb. (4 cups) GREEN BEANS
1 tsp. chopped ONION**
2 Tbsp. OLIVE OIL
1/4 cup COTTAGE CHEESE
1/4 cup diced CELERY
1 tsp. minced GREEN PEPPER
1 tsp. SUGAR

Cook beans in boiling water (or steam or microwave), until tender; drain if any water remains. Cook celery, onion and green pepper until soft and yellow; add to hot beans. Add sugar and salt to taste. Heat. Top with cottage cheese.

SERVING SIZE: 1/2 cup

CALORIES: 82    CHOL. 2 mg.    FAT: 5 g.    SODIUM: 42 mg.

* = Dangerous to Some    ** = Consume with Caution    (see Pages 22 & 23)

# Italian Steamed Artichokes

**Quick and Easy**
**Makes 1 serving**

*If you've never tried artichokes, try this low-calorie, easy dish.*

1 large ARTICHOKE (about 1 lb.)
1 BAY LEAF
1/2 tsp. DRIED OREGANO
1 GARLIC CLOVE, sliced thin
1/4 tsp. CORIANDER SEEDS
1/2 tsp. DRIED BASIL

Snip the thorns off the artichoke leaves. Place the garlic slices inside the leaves throughout the artichoke. Put the artichoke into a medium-size saucepan. Add water to come halfway up the artichoke. Put the bay leaf in the water; crush the coriander seeds, oregano and basil together; sprinkle on top of the artichoke. Cook over medium heat for 30 minutes or until the leaves pull off easily.

SERVING SIZE: 1 artichoke

CALORIES: 44     CHOL.: 0     FAT: 0     SODIUM: 30 mg.

# Minted Citrus Carrots

**Quick and Easy**
**Prepare Ahead**
**Makes 4 servings**          **\*\*Orange juice, lemon juice**

*The mint especially makes these carrots different. The sauce can also be served on hot, cooked carrots.*

Juice of medium ORANGE\*\*
1/4 cup freshly chopped MINT
3 large CARROTS, peeled and shredded
Juice of 1 medium LEMON\*\*
1/8 tsp. GROUND PEPPER

In small bowl, whisk juices, mint and pepper together. Toss with shredded carrots and refrigerate. Serve cold.

SERVING SIZE: 1/2 cup

CALORIES: 52     CHOL.: 0     FAT: 0     SODIUM: 36 mg.

\* = Dangerous to Some   \*\* = Consume with Caution   (see Pages 22 & 23)

# Lemon-Garlic Asparagus

**Quick and Easy**

**Makes 4 servings**          **\*\*Onion, lemon rind and lemon juice**

*A tasty method for preparing asparagus; use microwave if preferred.*

1 lb. fresh ASPARAGUS SPEARS
1 CLOVE GARLIC, crushed
1/2 tsp. THYME
1/2 tsp. BLACK PEPPER
1 cup LOW-SODIUM CHICKEN BROTH (or use CHICKEN
    BOUILLON and water)
1 medium ONION**, sliced
1 tsp. grated LEMON RIND**
1 BAY LEAF
2 Tbsp. LEMON JUICE**

Wash asparagus in cold water. Break off tough ends. Combine rest of the ingredients in a saucepan. Cover and simmer 15 minutes, then remove bay leaf. Add asparagus. Cover and simmer just until asparagus is tender.

SERVING SIZE: 1/2 cup

CALORIES: 42    CHOL. : 0    FAT: 0    SODIUM: 4 mg.

---

\* = Dangerous to Some    \*\* = Consume with Caution    (see Pages 22 & 23)

# Lemon-Herb Twice Baked Potatoes

Quick and Easy
Prepare Ahead
**Onion, lemon peel

**Makes 6 servings**

*These popular stuffed baked potatoes have become almost a staple in American diets. They can be prepared ahead of time and successfully reheated.*

1/3 cup chopped ONION**
1 CLOVE GARLIC, minced
1/2 cup hot SKIM MILK
1/8 tsp. GROUND WHITE PEPPER
1 Tbsp. chopped FRESH DILL or 1 tsp. DILL WEED
6 small BAKING POTATOES (4 to 6 oz. each)
2 Tbsp. MARGARINE
1 tsp. grated LEMON PEEL**
1 Tbsp. finely chopped PARSLEY
PAPRIKA

Bake potatoes at 400 degrees until done, about 45 minutes. Let stand at room temperature until cool enough to handle.

Meanwhile, sauté onion and garlic in margarine until tender; set aside.

Cut a slice from the top of each potato; scoop out the insides, being careful not to break skins. Mash potato insides; beat in prepared onion mixture, hot skim milk, lemon peel and pepper. Mix in dill weed and parsley.

Arrange potato skins in a baking dish; pile mashed potato mixture into skins; sprinkle with paprika. Bake at 400 degrees for 30 minutes or until lightly brown.

MICROWAVE: Pierce potatoes with fork; place 1 inch apart on paper toweling in microwave oven; microwave on HIGH (100% power) for 15 to 17 minutes or until tender, turning over and rearranging after 10 minutes.

In 1-quart microwave-proof glass measure, melt margarine

(Continued on next page)

* = Dangerous to Some   ** = Consume with Caution   (see Pages 22 & 23)

(Continued from previous page)

on HIGH for 1/2 to 1 minute. Add onion and garlic. Microwave on HIGH for 1 minute.

Continue assembling potatoes as above. Arrange in a 9-inch microwave-proof pie plate. Microwave on HIGH for 4 to 5 minutes or until heated through, rearranging after 2 minutes.

SERVING SIZE: 1 stuffed potato

CALORIES: 150    CHOL.: 0    FAT: 4 g.    SODIUM: 53 mg.

# Mexican Corn

**Quick and Easy**
**Makes 4 servings**

*A colorful way to serve frozen corn, or off-the-cob fresh corn.*

**1 (10 oz.) pkg. frozen WHOLE KERNEL GOLDEN CORN**
**1 CLOVE GARLIC, crushed**
**1 Tbsp. PIMENTO pieces or, chopped RED BELL PEPPERS**
**2 Tbsp. MARGARINE**
**1/2 cup chopped GREEN PEPPER**
**dash GROUND BLACK PEPPER**
**WARM WATER**

Melt margarine in a saucepan over medium heat. Stir in corn, green pepper, garlic and pepper. Cover and simmer for 10 minutes, stirring occasionally. Mix in pimento and continue cooking 2 minutes or until corn is tender. If necessary, stir in a little warm water to prevent sticking. Serve hot.

MICROWAVE: In a 1-1/2 quart microwave-proof casserole, microwave margarine on HIGH (100% power) for 40 to 45 seconds. Add corn, green pepper, garlic, black pepper and pimento. Cover; microwave on HIGH for 4 to 5 minutes, stirring once. Stir before serving.

SERVING SIZE: 1/2 cup

CALORIES: 117    CHOL.: 0    FAT: 6 g.    SODIUM: 51 mg.

* = Dangerous to Some    ** = Consume with Caution    (see Pages 22 & 23)

# New Potatoes in Lemon Parsley Sauce

**Makes 2 servings**

**Quick and Easy**
**\*\*Lemon peel, lemon juice**

*The lemon peel and chopped parsley add interest to the wonderful flavor of new potatoes.*

4 NEW POTATOES (about 1/2 lb.)
1 Tbsp. LEMON JUICE\*\*
1/2 tsp. grated LEMON PEEL\*\*
1 Tbsp. MARGARINE
1 Tbsp. chopped PARSLEY
BOILING WATER

Cook potatoes in boiling water for 15 to 20 minutes or until tender.  Drain, peel and quarter (if desired).

Melt margarine in saucepan over low heat; mix in lemon peel, lemon juice and parsley.  Add potatoes and cook over medium heat, turning frequently, until hot and coated with margarine.

MICROWAVE:  In 1-quart microwave-proof casserole, cover and microwave potatoes and 1/4 cup water on HIGH (100% power) for 5 to 7 minutes.  Drain, peel and quarter potatoes, if desired.  In same dish, microwave margarine on HIGH for 30 seconds.  Add lemon peel, lemon juice, parsley and potatoes.  Microwave on HIGH for 30 seconds.  Toss potatoes to coat with margarine before serving.

SERVING SIZE:  2 new potatoes (4 ounces)

CALORIES: 142    CHOL.: 0    FAT: 6 g.    SODIUM: 57 mg.

* = Dangerous to Some    \*\* = Consume with Caution    (see Pages 22 & 23)

# Oriental Spinach

**Makes 3 servings**

Quick and Easy
**Soy sauce

1 CLOVE GARLIC, crushed
1 lb. FRESH SPINACH, washed and drained (tough portions
    of stem removed), large leaves cut in pieces
1 tsp. WHITE VINEGAR
1/2 tsp. SOY SAUCE**
1/4 tsp. POWDERED GINGER
1-1/2 Tbsp. WATER
NON-STICK VEGETABLE SPRAY
SWEETENER to taste

Mix all sauce ingredients and set aside. Spray wok or frying pan with cooking spray. Heat; add garlic. Stir-fry 10 seconds. Add spinach and stir-fry 1 minute or until wilted. Add sauce mixture, stir and serve.

SERVING SIZE: 1/2 cup

CALORIES: 41    CHOL.: 0    FAT: 0.5 g.    SODIUM: 165 mg.

# Parsley Potato Cakes

**Quick and Easy**
**Makes 6 servings**

*Everyone seems to like potato patties.*

4 cups MASHED
    POTATOES, cold
2 Tbsp. OLIVE OIL
1/4 cup PARSLEY, chopped
1/2 tsp. GARLIC POWDER
1/2 tsp. MUSTARD POWDER
MARGARINE, melted, as
    needed, or spray
FLOUR, as needed

Combine potatoes, oil, parsley, mustard and garlic powders in large bowl. Mix well; form mixture into patties. Dip patties in flour; shake off excess. Heat margarine or spray; add patties. Cook over medium heat until golden brown on both sides.

SERVING SIZE: one 2/3 cup patty

CALORIES: 252    CHOL.: 18 mg.    FAT: 16 g.    SODIUM: 474 mg.

* = Dangerous to Some    ** = Consume with Caution    (see Pages 22 & 23)

# Peas Superb

**Makes 5 servings**

*A delicious way to serve peas; frozen peas also work well, but shorten the cooking time. If microwaving, stir frozen peas into mushroom mixture.*

**2-1/2 cups FRESH PEAS (about 2 lbs., unshelled)**
**1 cup sliced fresh MUSHROOMS***
**1 Tbsp. MARGARINE**
**2 Tbsp. chopped ONION****
**BOILING WATER**

Cook peas in a small amount of boiling water until tender. Melt margarine in large skillet. Add mushrooms and onion and sauté until tender; add peas and cook until heated through. Serve immediately.

MICROWAVE: In 1-quart microwave-proof bowl, cover and microwave peas and 1/4 cup water on HIGH (100% power) for 7 to 8 minutes, stirring after 4 minutes. Drain; set aside.

In 1-quart microwave-proof casserole, microwave margarine on HIGH for 30 seconds, stir in mushrooms and onions. Microwave on HIGH for 1 minute. Stir in peas; microwave on HIGH for 2 to 3 minutes, stirring after 1-1/2 minutes. Stir before serving.

SERVING SIZE: 1/2 cup

CALORIES: 88     CHOL.: 0     FAT: 3 g.     SODIUM: 24 mg.

* = Dangerous to Some   ** = Consume with Caution   (see Pages 22 & 23)

# Potato Pancakes

**Makes 1 dozen pancakes, 6 servings**

Quick and Easy
**Onion

*Potato pancakes made with raw potatoes are extra-flavorful (especially if you have equipment to cube the potatoes!) White pepper not only looks more attractive with white foods, but tastes different, too.*

1/2 cup EGG SUBSTITUTE, or 2 EGGS
1/2 cup coarsely chopped ONION**
1/8 tsp. GROUND WHITE PEPPER
3 cups raw POTATOES, cubed
1/4 cup ALL-PURPOSE FLOUR
2 Tbsp. MARGARINE
APPLESAUCE

Place egg substitute in blender container; add potatoes, onion, flour and pepper. Blend until cubes are well grated and the mixture is evenly rough in consistency.

Melt 1 teaspoon margarine on hot griddle for every 2 pancakes. For each pancake, pour 1/4 cup batter onto hot griddle. Fry on both sides until well browned, about 3 minutes per side. Serve hot with applesauce, if desired.

SERVING SIZE: 2 small pancakes

CALORIES: 125    CHOL.: 0    FAT: 4 g.    SODIUM: 63 mg.

* = Dangerous to Some    ** = Consume with Caution    (see Pages 22 & 23)

# Roasted Garlic Potatoes

**Makes 6 servings**

Easy
**Onion

*These crusty potatoes are a favorite of many, with their crunchy surface and tender interior. Potatoes also are one of the nation's largest source of vitamin C.*

1/4 cup OLIVE OIL
1 lb. RED POTATOES
2 Tbsp. GARLIC, minced
1 medium ONION**, sliced

Preheat oven to 375 degrees. Heat oil in skillet. Add onions and garlic. Sauté until just golden. Cut potatoes into wedges; add to skillet. Sauté until golden brown and well coated. Transfer to baking pan; bake until dark golden brown and fork tender, about 20 minutes.

SERVING SIZE: 1/2 cup

CALORIES: 150    CHOL.: 0    FAT: 9 g.    SODIUM: 7 mg.

# Steamed Spring Asparagus

Easy
**Makes 6 servings**

*Serve with creamed tuna or chicken for lunch or supper.*

1/4 cup SUGAR
1 lb. SPRING ASPARAGUS, trimmed
1/2 stick BUTTER (1/4 cup)
1 quart BOILING WATER
SALT and PEPPER to taste

Heat heavy saucepan. Add sugar; stir just until melted. Add asparagus and boiling water. Cover pan; boil hard for 5 minutes. Drain. Melt butter; add asparagus; stir just until well coated and hot. Season to taste.

SERVING SIZE: 1/2 cup

CALORIES: 94    CHOL.: 22 mg.  FAT: 8 g.  SODIUM: 83 mg.

* = Dangerous to Some   ** = Consume with Caution   (see Pages 22 & 23)

# Sweet Potatoes a la Orange

**Makes 8 servings**

Easy
**Dried apricots, orange

2 lbs. SWEET POTATOES, cooked, or 2 pounds
    canned SWEET POTATOES
2 Tbsp. MARGARINE, melted
Fresh ORANGE slices**
16 DRIED APRICOT halves**
1/2 tsp. GROUND CINNAMON
SWEETENER to taste

Arrange the sweet potatoes in a shallow baking dish. Combine the margarine and cinnamon. Pour over potatoes. Arrange the apricot halves on top. Cover the dish and bake at 425 degrees for about 15 minutes. Add sweetener, if desired. Add orange slices and serve.

SERVING SIZE: 2/3 cup

CALORIES: 185   CHOL.: 0   FAT: 7 g.   SODIUM: 79 mg.


# Vegetable Melange

**Makes 2 servings**

Quick and Easy
**Onion

*Save out a few of these vegetables from your raw vegetable purchases for a colorful combination of flavors.*

1 small ZUCCHINI, shredded
2 CARROTS, shredded
1 small YELLOW SQUASH,
    shredded

1 small ONION**, sliced
    thin
2 Tbsp. WATER
2 tsp. MARGARINE

Combine the zucchini, yellow squash, carrots, onion and water in a skillet. Cover and cook over medium heat for 4 to 5 minutes, or until vegetables are tender. Add margarine. Sauté, uncovered until all moisture has evaporated. Serve immediately.

SERVING SIZE: 1/2 cup

CALORIES: 94   CHOL.: 0   FAT: 4 g.   SODIUM: 83 mg.

* = Dangerous to Some   ** = Consume with Caution   (see Pages 22 & 23)

# Wild Rice Casserole

**Makes 6 servings**

*A great way to serve crunchy rice. Can be prepared the day before and reheated for a party. Delicious served with poultry. All brown rice works fine, too.*

1/2 cup **WILD RICE**
1/2 cup **BROWN RICE**
1 cup **MEDIUM WHITE SAUCE** (or 1 cup undiluted **MUSHROOM SOUP***)
1 box (4 oz.) **MUSHROOMS*** cut up (or 1 small can **MUSHROOMS***)
1 large **ONION****, chopped
1 cup **WATER**
**COOKING SPRAY**

Clean wild rice by first putting it in a separate bowl of water, picking out hulls, etc.; drain. Cook all rice with the 1 cup of water, at low temperature, in tightly covered pan for about 1/2 hour. Don't let it get mushy.

In the meantime, brown mushroom pieces and onion until slightly cooked—still crunchy.

Stir white sauce or mushroom soup, rice and onion-mushroom mixture together with a fork, only until lightly combined. Place in greased casserole—to be baked later, or if serving, bake 25 minutes at 350 degrees.

SERVING SIZE: 2/3 cup

CALORIES: 90    CHOL.: 0    FAT: 1 g.    SODIUM: 400 mg.

* = Dangerous to Some    ** = Consume with Caution    (see Pages 22 & 23)

# Yellow Squash Fritters

**Quick and Easy**
**\*\*Onion**

**Makes 1 serving**

*Always save (or drink now) the drained water from vegetables. this liquid has much of the water-soluble vitamins.*

1 cup steamed, diced YELLOW SQUASH, well drained
1 EGG, or 1/4 cup EGG SUBSTITUTE
1 slice BREAD, crumbled
1 tsp. PARSLEY FLAKES
1 tsp. DRIED ONION FLAKES**
NON-STICK VEGETABLE SPRAY

In blender combine all ingredients and blend just until squash is finely chopped. Drop by tablespoons onto sprayed griddle. Cook over moderate heat until browned on bottom. Turn and cook until top is browned.

SERVING SIZE: 1 fritter

CALORIES: 182  CHOL.: 0 mg.  FAT: 2 g. SODIUM: 80 mg.

# Zucchini Sauté

**Quick and Easy**
**\*Mushrooms**
**\*\*Onion**

**Makes 8 servings**

*A nice change from "just zucchini"*

1 Tbsp. MARGARINE
3 medium ZUCCHINI, thinly sliced
1 cup sliced fresh MUSHROOMS*
2 CLOVES GARLIC, minced
1 small GREEN PEPPER, coarsely chopped
1/8 tsp. GROUND BLACK PEPPER

Melt margarine in large skillet over medium heat. Add zucchini, green pepper and garlic. Sauté until zucchini is tender and crisp, about 5 minutes. Add mushrooms and pepper, cook and stir about 5 minutes more until vegetables are tender but firm.

SERVING SIZE: 1/2 cup

CALORIES: 27    CHOL.: 0    FAT: 2 g.    SODIUM: 14 mg.

* = Dangerous to Some   ** = Consume with Caution   (see Pages 22 & 23)

# Sauces, Toppings
## and your own Pizza Base!

# Pizza Party Base

**Prepare Ahead**

**Makes 2 (14-inch) pizzas, 8 slices per pie**

*Everyone will be impressed with the fact that you can make your own pizza base. Biscuit dough can substitute effectively, too—rolled to 1/8" thickness because it rises so much.*

**2-3/4 to 3-1/4 cups ALL-PURPOSE FLOUR**
**1/8 tsp. GROUND BLACK PEPPER**
**1 cup WATER**
**2 cups LOW-SODIUM TOMATO JUICE**
**3/4 cup (6 cubes) frozen *LOW-SODIUM TOMATO BASE* (see page 165) or *TOMATO FRESH SALSA* (see page 164)**
**1/2 tsp. crushed fresh GARLIC**
**1 Tbsp. SUGAR**
**1 pkg. ACTIVE DRY YEAST**
**1/4 cup MARGARINE**
**1 tsp. OREGANO LEAVES**

Mix 1 cup flour, sugar and undissolved yeast. Heat margarine and water in a saucepan until very warm (120 to 130 degrees). Margarine does not need to melt. Gradually add to dry ingredients and beat 2 minutes at medium speed of electric mixer, scraping bowl occasionally; add 1/2 cup flour. Beat at high speed 2 minutes, scraping bowl occasionally.

Stir in enough additional flour to make a stiff dough. Turn out onto a floured board; knead until smooth and elastic, about 4 to 5 minutes. Place in a greased bowl, turning to grease top. Cover; let rise in a warm draft-free place until doubled in size, about 1 hour.

Combine tomato juice, Tomato Base, oregano, garlic and pepper in a medium saucepan. Bring to a boil over medium high heat, stirring occasionally. Reduce heat to low and simmer until reduced to 1-1/2 cups.

Punch dough down; divide in half. Shape each half into a ball; cover and let stand 10 minutes. Roll and stretch each half to a 14-inch circle. Place in 2 greased 14-inch pizza pans,

(Continued on next page)

* = Dangerous to Some   ** = Consume with Caution   (see Pages 22 & 23)

forming a standing rim of dough around edges.

Spread half of prepared tomato sauce over each crust and top pies with either **Vegetable Topping** *(see page 164)* or **Beef and Zucchini Topping** *(see below)*. Bake at 375 degrees for 20 to 25 minutes or until done.

NOTE: If desired, pizza crust can be prebaked at 375 degrees for 7 minutes and frozen. When ready to use, defrost crust; top and bake as directed above.

Nutritional value included in recipes using pizza crust.

# Beef and Zucchini Topping

Quick and Easy

**Makes 8 servings on one 14-inch pizza crust (with tomato sauce or cottage cheese).**

*Vary a pizza with this different topping; also can be used on stuffed baked potatoes or tortillas.*

**1 Tbsp. MARGARINE**
**1/4 lb. lean GROUND BEEF**
**1 cup sliced ZUCCHINI**

Melt margarine in skillet over medium heat. Saute sliced zucchini until tender crisp, about 2 to 3 minutes. Remove from pan. Crumble and brown ground beef in skillet over medium heat. Remove from skillet and drain well.

Arrange beef and zucchini on pizza crust and bake as directed. (see **Party Pizza Base**)

SERVING SIZE: 1/8 pizza

CALORIES: 174   CHOL.: 9 mg.   FAT: 6 g.   SODIUM: 97 mg.

* = Dangerous to Some   ** = Consume with Caution   (see Pages 22 & 23)

# Vegetable Topping

**Easy**
***Mushrooms**
****Onion**

**Makes 8 servings on 14-inch pizza crust**

*Another topping for pizza.*

1 Tbsp. MARGARINE
3/4 cup thinly sliced GREEN PEPPER strips
2 cups sliced MUSHROOMS*
3/4 cup thinly sliced ONION**

Melt margarine in skillet over medium heat. Saute sliced mushrooms until slightly golden. Remove from heat. Toss in green pepper strips and sliced onion. Arrange topping on a 14-inch pizza crust and bake as directed. (see **Party Pizza Base**)

SERVING SIZE: 1/8 pizza

CALORIES: 165   CHOL.: 5 mg.   FAT: 5 g.   SODIUM: 94 mg.

# Tomato Fresh Salsa

**Prepare Ahead**
****Onion, lemon juice**

**Makes 4-1/2 cups salsa**

*This salsa has many uses; try it with tortilla or corn chips.*

3-1/2 cups (28 oz. can) CRUSHED TOMATOES
1/2 cup (4 oz.) diced GREEN CHILES
1/2 cup sliced GREEN ONIONS**, tops included
1/3 cup fresh LEMON JUICE**
1/4 tsp. RED PEPPER FLAKES (optional)
1-1/2 tsp. GARLIC SALT
2 Tbsp. finely chopped fresh CILANTRO or PARSLEY
2 tsp. DRIED OREGANO LEAVES, crushed
1/2 tsp. GROUND CUMIN

In large bowl, combine tomatoes, diced green chiles, green onion, lemon juice, cilantro or parsley, oregano, garlic salt, cumin and red pepper flakes, if desired. Mix well. Cover and refrigerate for 4 hours to allow flavors to blend.

SERVING SIZE: 1 tablespoon

CALORIES: 14   CHOL.: 0      FAT: 0      SODIUM: 262 mg.

* = Dangerous to Some    ** = Consume with Caution    (see Pages 22 & 23)

# Low-Sodium Tomato Base

**Makes 3 cups (24 cubes)**

Prepare Ahead
**Onion

*This on-hand tomato base adds its own special flavor to every dish that includes it.*

**5 lbs. ripe TOMATOES, coarsely chopped**
**1 cup grated CARROTS**
**1 cup chopped ONIONS****
**1 cup minced RED PEPPER**

Combine tomatoes, onions, carrots and pepper in large heavy pan. Cover; cook over medium-high heat, stirring occasionally, until tomatoes are a liquid and pulp mixture, about 30 minutes. Uncover; cook over medium heat, stirring occasionally, until thickened and reduced by half, about 3-1/2 to 4 hours. Put mixture through a sieve to remove skins and seeds.

Place sieved mixture in a medium saucepan. Partially cover and cook over medium heat until very thick, making about 3 cups. Cool.

Measure 2 tablespoons tomato base into individual ice cube tray sections. Freeze until firm. Remove from trays and store in a plastic bag or lidded container. Use as directed in recipes.

SERVING SIZE: 1 cube (2 tablespoons)

CALORIES: 23     CHOL.: 0     FAT: 0     SODIUM: 9 mg.

* = Dangerous to Some   ** = Consume with Caution   (see Pages 22 & 23)

# Easy Tomato Sauce

*A marinara-type spaghetti sauce—the type Italian wives
rushed to make when they first saw their sailor-husbands'
ships appear homeward bound on the horizon.*

2 tsp. OLIVE OIL
2 CLOVES GARLIC, minced
2 tsp. minced FRESH OREGANO
1/8 to 1/4 tsp. PEPPER
1/2 cup finely chopped ONION**
2 (28 oz.) cans ITALIAN TOMATOES, undrained and
    chopped
1/4 cup chopped FRESH BASIL

Heat oil in a large skillet over medium-low heat until hot.
Add onion, and saute until tender. Add garlic; saute 1 minute.
Stir in tomatoes, and bring to a boil. Add remaining ingredients; stir well. Reduce heat to medium-low and cook, uncovered, until thickened, stirring frequently. Serve over cooked
pasta.

Variation: Fiery Tomato and Red Pepper Sauce: add 1/4
teaspoon crushed red pepper to basil, oregano and black pepper.

SERVING SIZE: 1/2 cup

CALORIES: 56    CHOL.: 0    FAT: 1.6 g.    SODIUM: 324 mg.

---

* = Dangerous to Some    ** = Consume with Caution    (see Pages 22 & 23)

# Classic Iowa Barbecue Sauce

**Quick and Easy**
***Worcestershire sauce**

**Makes 2/3 cup sauce**
****Orange juice**

*A barbecue sauce that can be used on any meat, fish or poultry. The orange juice is the mystery ingredient.*

1/2 cup CATSUP
1 CLOVE GARLIC, minced or 1/4 tsp. GARLIC POWDER
1 Tbsp. ORANGE JUICE CONCENTRATE**
2 Tbsp. PREPARED MUSTARD
1 Tbsp. WHITE VINEGAR
1 Tbsp. WORCESTERSHIRE SAUCE*

Combine all ingredients. Spread over meat 4 minutes prior to removing from grill. Grill on one side for 2 minutes. Turn meat, coat the other side and grill for an additional 2 minutes.

SERVING SIZE: 1 tablespoon

CALORIES: 40    CHOL.: 0    FAT: 1 g.  SODIUM: 532 mg.


# Green Onion Potato Topping

**Quick and Easy**
***Mayonnaise**

**Makes 1 cup**
****Green onions**

1 cup cholesterol-free REDUCED CALORIE MAYONNAISE*
    (check label)
1/4 cup sliced GREEN ONIONS**

Combine ingredients in a small bowl. Serve over baked potato.

SERVING SIZE: 1 tablespoon

CALORIES: 50    CHOL.: 0    FAT: 3 g.  SODIUM: 80 mg.


* = Dangerous to Some   ** = Consume with Caution   (see Pages 22 & 23)

# Tomato and Mushroom Sauce

**Prepare Ahead**
***Mushrooms**

**Makes 4 cups**                                ****Onion**

*Another spaghetti sauce to prepare ahead of time. Add a pinch of sugar or sweetener to taste, as your grandmother used to for added flavor.*

**2 tsp. OLIVE OIL**
**2 CLOVES GARLIC, minced**
**2 tsp. minced fresh OREGANO**
**1/8 to 1/4 tsp. PEPPER**
**2 cups chopped fresh MUSHROOMS***
**1/2 cup finely chopped ONION****
**2 (28 oz.) cans ITALIAN TOMATOES, undrained and**
    **chopped**
**1/4 cup chopped FRESH BASIL**

Heat oil in a large skillet over medium-low heat until hot. Add onion, and saute until tender. Add garlic; saute 1 minute. Add mushrooms to sauteed onion mixture. Stir in tomatoes and bring to a boil. Add remaining ingredients and stir well. Reduce heat to medium-low and cook, uncovered, 1-1/2 hours or until thickened, stirring frequently.

SERVING SIZE: 1/2 cup

CALORIES: 61     CHOL.: 0     FAT: 1.7 g.     SODIUM: 325 mg.

---

# Sauce Dijonnaise

**Makes about 2/3 cup**

Quick and Easy
**\*\*Lemon juice**

*Change the taste of plain vegetables with this sauce.*

1/2 cup light, regular, or unsalted MARGARINE
1 Tbsp. DIJON MUSTARD
1 Tbsp. LEMON JUICE\*\*
1/2 tsp. TARRAGON LEAVES

Melt margarine in small saucepan over medium heat. Whisk in lemon juice, mustard and tarragon. Serve over hot cooked vegetables.

SERVING SIZE: 1 tablespoon

Regular Margarine
CALORIES: 82    CHOL.: 0     FAT: 9 g.  SODIUM: 121 mg.
Unsalted Margarine
CALORIES: 82    CHOL.: 0     FAT: 9 g.  SODIUM: 45 mg.
Light Spread
CALORIES: 42    CHOL.: 0     FAT: 5 g.  SODIUM: 125 mg.

# Skinny-Dip Tartar Sauce

**Makes 1-1/4 cups**

Quick and Easy
**\*\*Yogurt, onion**

*This low-cal tartar sauce will spice up any seafood entree.*

3/4 cup LOW-FAT COTTAGE CHEESE
1/4 cup PLAIN NOFAT YOGURT\*\*
1 Tbsp. minced, fresh PARSLEY
1 Tbsp. chopped ONION\*\*
2 Tbsp. grated CUCUMBER
1 tsp. CELERY FLAKES
1/2 tsp. CAPERS, or to taste

Blend cottage cheese in blender until smooth. Mix in all other ingredients and refrigerate. Use within 2 days.

SERVING SIZE: 1 tablespoon

CALORIES: 12    CHOL.: 1 mg.  FAT: Trace  SODIUM: 25 mg.

* = Dangerous to Some   \*\* = Consume with Caution   (see Pages 22 & 23)

# Vegetable Relish

Makes 4 servings

**Prepare Ahead**
**\*\*Onion**

*This is the relish often seen in buffet or cafeteria serving lines.*

1 cup shredded CARROTS
1/2 cup chopped RED PEPPER
1/4 cup finely chopped RED ONION\*\*
1 tsp. SUGAR
1 Tbsp. VEGETABLE OIL
1 cup chopped CUCUMBERS
1/2 cup chopped GREEN PEPPER
3 Tbsp. WHITE VINEGAR
1/4 tsp. SALT

Combine carrot, cucumber, pepper and onion in a medium bowl. Set aside. Mix vinegar, sugar and salt together. Add oil and whisk thoroughly. Pour over vegetables and toss to coat. Cover and refrigerate for at least 1 hour before serving.

SERVING SIZE: 3/4 cup

CALORIES: 84     CHOL.: 0     FAT: 4 g.     SODIUM: 162 mg.

# Festive Cranberry Sauce

Makes 4 servings

**Quick and Easy**
**\*\*Orange**

*Turkey, especially, seems more festive with cranberry sauce and this one is tasty, yet different.*

2 cups fresh CRANBERRIES
1/4 cup WATER
1 cup frozen unsweetened STRAWBERRIES, defrosted
1 ORANGE\*\*, peeled and chopped
1 Tbsp. ARTIFICIAL SWEETENER

Put cranberries, orange and water in medium saucepan. Simmer until cranberries "pop". Remove from heat. Add sweetener to taste, plus strawberries. Chill and serve.

SERVING SIZE: 1/2 cup

CALORIES: 63     CHOL.: 0     FAT: 0     SODIUM: 1 mg.

* = Dangerous to Some     ** = Consume with Caution     (see Pages 22 & 23)

# Pear Butter

**Makes 6 cups**

*This treat is a great topping for toast or ice cream, or even tastes good with meat dishes.*

3-1/2 lb. PEARS, peeled and quartered (8 pears)
12 pkg. SWEETENER
2-1/2 tsp. VANILLA EXTRACT*
1/2 cup MARGARINE
1/3 cup LEMON JUICE** (2 lemons)

Mix pears and lemon juice in a saucepan. Bring to a boil. Cook covered over very low heat for 15 minutes, or until pears are tender. Drain well and reserve juice.

In another pan, bring juice to a boil and reduce to 1/4 cup (by evaporation). Blend pears in food processor or blender, add hot juice, margarine (if using a stick, sliced into sections) and vanilla. Blend until margarine is dissolved into pear mixture. Cool. Stir in sweetener. Pour pear butter in freezer bags or plastic freezer containers and refrigerate. (Pear butter will stay fresh in the refrigerator for about one week; freeze the extra pear butter that will be used later.)

SERVING SIZE: 1 tablespoon

CALORIES: 19    CHOL.: 0    FAT: 1 g.    SODIUM: 11 mg.

* = Dangerous to Some    ** = Consume with Caution    (see Pages 22 & 23)

# Lois' Cranberry Conserve

**Prepare Ahead-—Gourmet**

**Makes 1 quart to 5 cups**        **\*\*Pecans, orange, raisins**

*Just about the most-special cranberry accompaniment ever made. So good it's sometimes given as a gift for Thanksgiving or Christmas.*

**4 cups CRANBERRIES**
**1 cup nuts (PECANS\*\*—cut up, just broken)**
**1 small ORANGE\*\*, put through grater or blender**
**2-1/2 cups SUGAR**
**1 cup WATER**
**1 cup whole seedless RAISINS\*\***

Cook cranberries in the 1 cup of water until they pop—should all be popped. Cool and put through blender and then sieve.

Bring strained cranberries and sugar to a boil, then add nuts, raisins and orange. Let simmer, then stand until cool.

Prepare a few days before; flavor will permeate. Serve cold.

SERVING SIZE: 2 tablespoons

CALORIES: 75     CHOL.: 0     FAT: Trace     SODIUM: 30 mg.

\* = Dangerous to Some    \*\* = Consume with Caution    (see Pages 22 & 23)

# Breads, Muffins & Breakfasts

# Crunchy Bread Sticks

**Makes 8 bread sticks**

**Quick and Easy**
**\*\*Onion powder**

*Adding a bread variation to a meal can make it special;*
*poppy seeds could be used also.*

**2 Tbsp. MARGARINE**
**1/2 tsp. DRIED DILL WEED**
**2 slices WHITE BREAD**
**dash ONION POWDER\*\***

Melt margarine and mix in dill weed and onion powder. Trim crust from bread and brush both sides of slices with margarine mixture. Cut each slice into 4 strips. Set on an ungreased baking sheet and bake at 350 degrees for 12 to 15 minutes, turning once, or until golden brown and crisp.

**Sesame Sticks:** Substitute 2 tablespoons sesame seed for dill weed and onion powder.

SERVING SIZE: 1 bread stick

**Crunchy Bread Sticks**
CALORIES: 41    CHOL.: 0    FAT: 3 g.   SODIUM: 54 mg.

**Sesame Sticks**
CALORIES: 54    CHOL.: 0    FAT: 4 g.   SODIUM: 54 mg.

* = Dangerous to Some    ** = Consume with Caution    (see Pages 22 & 23)

# Date-and-Nut Bread

**Makes 1 loaf**

**Prepare Ahead—Gourmet**
**\*Vanilla extract**
**\*\*Walnuts, pecans, dates**

*With this very special sliced bread in the freezer, you'll always be ready for drop-in guests. It stays moist and wonderful, frozen, even up to one year! Makes a meal special; great addition as a small sandwich (with cream cheese or margarine) and ready to eat; can be prepared ahead of time, too.*

**3/4 cup chopped WALNUTS\*\* or PECANS\*\***
**1-1/2 tsp. BAKING SODA**
**1-1/2 cups sifted ALL-PURPOSE FLOUR**
**3 Tbsp. SHORTENING**
**1 cup cut-up, pitted DATES\*\***
**3/4 cup boiling WATER**
**2 EGGS or 1/2 cup EGG SUBSTITUTE**
**1 tsp. VANILLA\***
**1/2 tsp. SALT**
**1 cup GRANULATED SUGAR**

With fork, mix walnuts, dates, soda, salt. Add shortening, water; let stand 20 minutes. Start heating oven to 350 degrees. Grease 9 x 5 x 3-inch loaf pan. With fork, beat eggs; beat in vanilla, sugar, flour. Mix in date mixture until just blended; turn into pan. Bake 1 hour, 5 minutes, or until loaf tests baked. Cool in pan 10 minutes; remove. Cool overnight before slicing. Freezes beautifully!

SERVING SIZE: 1 slice (3/16 inch)

CALORIES: 124  CHOL.: 0.2 mg.  FAT: 2.4 g. SODIUM: 128 mg.

* = Dangerous to Some   ** = Consume with Caution   (see Pages 22 & 23)

# Low-Salt Challah

**Makes 2 loaves, 18 slices per loaf**        **Prepare Ahead**

*Try this yeast bread. The less flour used in kneading, the more tender the challah.*

**1 cup WARM WATER (105 to 115 degrees)**
**3/4 cup EGG SUBSTITUTE ( room temperature), or 3 EGGS**
**2 Tbsp. SUGAR**
**5-1/4 to 5-3/4 cups ALL-PURPOSE FLOUR**
**1/2 cup SWEET UNSALTED MARGARINE, melted and**
    **slightly cooled**
**1 pkg. ACTIVE DRY YEAST**
**2 tsp. EGG SUBSTITUTE**
**POPPY SEED**
**dash POWDERED SAFFRON, optional**

Measure warm water into large warm bowl. Sprinkle in yeast; stir until dissolved. Stir in sugar, saffron and margarine. Blend in 3/4 cup egg substitute; add 3 cups flour; beat until smooth. Stir in enough additional flour to form a stiff dough. Turn out onto a lightly floured board; knead until smooth and elastic, about 8 to 10 minutes. Place in a greased bowl, turning to grease top. Cover, let rise in warm draft-free place until doubled in size, about 1 hour.

Punch dough down; divide in half. Divide each half into 2 pieces, one about 1/3 of dough and the other about 2/3 of dough. Divide larger piece into 3 equal pieces. Roll each piece into a 12-inch rope. Braid the 3 ropes together; pinch ends to seal. Divide smaller piece into 3 equal pieces. Roll each piece into a 10-inch rope. Braid the ropes together; place on top of large braid. Seal braids together at ends. Repeat with remaining dough to form second loaf. Brush braids with 2 teaspoons egg substitute; sprinkle with poppy seed. Cover, let rise in warm draft-free place until doubled in size, about 1 hour.

Bake at 375 degrees for 20 to 25 minutes or until done. Remove from baking sheets and cool on wire racks.

SERVING SIZE: 1 slice

CALORIES: 97     CHOL.: 0     FAT: 3 g.     SODIUM: 8 mg.

---

* = Dangerous to Some    ** = Consume with Caution    (see Pages 22 & 23)

# Orange "Chocolate" Chip Bread

**Makes 16 servings**

**Prepare Ahead**
**\*\*Orange juice, orange peel,
buttermilk**

*The orange juice and peel surprisingly complement the carob
chips and vice versa.*

1/4 cup ORANGE JUICE**
1/3 cup SUGAR
1/2 cup CAROB CHIPS (semi-sweet kisses)
1 Tbsp. grated fresh ORANGE PEEL**
1 cup SKIM MILK
1 EGG, slightly beaten
3 cups BUTTERMILK** BISCUIT MIX

Heat oven to 350 degrees. Grease 9 x 5 x 2-3/4-inch loaf pan.
In a medium mixing bowl, combine milk, orange juice, sugar,
egg and orange peel; stir into baking mix. Beat until well
combined, about 1 minute. Stir in carob chips; pour into
prepared pan; bake 45 to 50 minutes or until wooden toothpick
inserted in center comes out clean. Cool 10 minutes; remove
from pan. Cool completely.

SERVING SIZE: one 1/2 inch slice

CALORIES: 161  CHOL.: 0 mg.  FAT: 10 g. SODIUM: 374 mg.

* = Dangerous to Some   ** = Consume with Caution   (see Pages 22 & 23)

# Pecan Sticky Buns

**Makes 18 buns**

Prepare Ahead<br>**Pecans

*Always a great favorite as you may have noticed in the shopping malls and at fairs.  Of course, if nuts are a trigger agent for headaches for you, skip the pecans.*

3-1/4 to 3-3/4 cups ALL-PURPOSE FLOUR
1/4 cup WATER
1/2 cup EGG SUBSTITUTE, or 2 EGGS
1/4 cup SUGAR
1/2 cup SKIM MILK
1/3 cup MARGARINE
1 pkg. ACTIVE DRY YEAST

For the topping and filling:

1-1/4 cup firmly packed DARK BROWN SUGAR
1/2 cup PECAN** pieces
6 Tbsp. MARGARINE
1/2 cup LIGHT CORN SYRUP

In large bowl, mix 1 cup flour, sugar and undissolved yeast. In saucepan, heat milk, water and 1/3 cup margarine to 120 to 130 degrees.  Margarine need not melt.  Add to dry ingredients and beat 2 minutes at medium speed of mixer, scraping bowl occasionally.  Add egg substitute and 1/2 cup flour.  Beat at high speed for 2 minutes.  Stir in enough additional flour to make a soft dough.

Knead on lightly floured board 8 to 10 minutes.  Place in greased bowl, turning to grease top.  Cover, let rise in warm draft-free place, until doubled, about 1 hour.

While dough is rising, prepare pan.  Mix 4 tablespoons margarine with 1 cup brown sugar and corn syrup.  Cook and stir until sugar dissolves.  Pour into greased 13 x 9 x 2-inch baking pan.  Sprinkle with pecan pieces.

Punch dough down; divide in half.  Roll each half to a 14 x 9-inch rectangle.  Melt remaining margarine and brush on dough; sprinkle with remaining brown sugar.  Roll up to form

* = Dangerous to Some    ** = Consume with Caution    (see Pages 22 & 23)

9-inch rolls. Pinch seams. Cut each roll into 9 slices. Arrange in prepared pan. Cover; let rise until doubled, about 45 minutes.

Bake at 375 degrees for 20 to 25 minutes or until done. Cool in pan for 5 minutes, then invert onto wire rack to cool completely.

SERVING SIZE: 1 bun

CALORIES: 274    CHOL.: 0    FAT: 9 g.    SODIUM: 83 mg.

# Pumpkin Bread

**Prepare Ahead**
**Gourmet**
**Makes 3 loaves**                    **\*\*Nuts, raisins**

*This moist, easy-to-make bread is a winner. It doesn't dry out nor pick up freezer-burn flavor. It's also easy to slice and won't crumble.*

| | |
|---|---|
| 3-1/2 cups FLOUR | 4 EGGS |
| 3 cups SUGAR | 2 cups canned PUMPKIN |
| 2 tsp. SODA | 1 cup chopped NUTS** |
| 2/3 cup WATER | 1 cup RAISINS** |
| 1 tsp. BAKING POWDER | 1 tsp. CINNAMON |
| 1-1/2 tsp. SALT | 1 tsp. NUTMEG |
| 1 cup OIL | |

Sift all dry ingredients together, including sugar, into a large mixing bowl. Make a well in the center, and add other ingredients, except raisins and nuts. Mix thoroughly. Add raisins and nuts, stir well.

Pour mixture into three greased and floured bread loaf pans and bake in preheated 350 degree oven for 1 hour. Let cool slightly before removing from pans. Wrap in foil (sliced), and store in the refrigerator. This bread may be frozen for up to 1 year.

SERVING SIZE: one 3/16 inch slice

CALORIES: 118    CHOL.: 0.1 mg. FAT: 3 g.    SODIUM: 126 mg.

* = Dangerous to Some    ** = Consume with Caution    (see Pages 22 & 23)

# Salt-Free Whole Wheat Bread

**Prepare Ahead**

**Makes 2 loaves, 15 slices per loaf**

*Whole wheat flour makes a closer-grained, less fluffy loaf because the whole wheat bran cuts the yeast-rising strands; close, solid structure compared to white bread.*

**4-1/2 to 5 cups ALL-PURPOSE FLOUR**
**2-1/4 cups WATER**
**1/4 cup HONEY**
**1/3 cup SWEET UNSALTED MARGARINE**
**2 cups WHOLE WHEAT FLOUR**
**1 Tbsp. SUGAR**
**2 pkgs. ACTIVE DRY YEAST**

Combine flours; in a large bowl thoroughly mix 2 cups flour mixture, sugar and undissolved yeast.

In saucepan, heat water, honey and margarine until very warm (120 to 130 degrees). Margarine does not need to melt. Gradually add to dry ingredients and beat 2 minutes at medium speed of electric mixer, scraping bowl occasionally. Stir in enough additional flour mixture to make a stiff dough. Turn out onto a lightly floured board and knead until smooth and elastic, about 8 to 10 minutes. Place in greased bowl, turning to grease top. Cover; let rise in warm draft-free place until doubled in size, about 40 minutes.

Punch dough down; turn out onto a lightly floured board. Divide dough in half. Shape each half into a loaf. Place in 2 greased 8-1/2 x 4-1/2 x 2-1/2-inch or 9 x 5 x 3-inch loaf pans. Cover; let rise in a warm draft-free place until doubled in size, about 45 minutes. Bake at 400 degrees for 30 to 35 minutes or until done. Remove from pans and cool on wire racks.

SERVING SIZE: 1 slice

CALORIES: 128    CHOL.: 0    FAT: 2 g.    SODIUM: 1 mg.

* = Dangerous to Some    ** = Consume with Caution    (see Pages 22 & 23)

# Soft Poppy Seed Loaf

**Makes 2 loaves (18 slices each)**

**Prepare Ahead**
***Vanilla and Almond extracts**
****Orange juice, orange peel**

*A delicious bread with its delicate almond, poppy seed, and orange flavors.*

1/2 tsp. SALT
3 cups FLOUR
2 tsp. VANILLA EXTRACT*
3/4 cup VEGETABLE OIL
1/2 cup FROZEN ORANGE JUICE CONCENTRATE**, thawed
2 Tbsp. POWDERED SUGAR
1-1/2 tsp. BAKING POWDER
1-1/2 cup SUGAR
1-1/2 cups SKIM MILK
1-1/2 tsp. ALMOND EXTRACT*
2 Tbsp. POPPY SEEDS
3/4 cup EGG SUBSTITUTE, or 3 EGGS
1 Tbsp. finely grated ORANGE PEEL**
NON-STICK VEGETABLE SPRAY

Combine all ingredients, except orange peel and powdered sugar, in a large mixing bowl. Beat for 2 minutes. Spray 2 loaf pans with non-stick vegetable cooking spray. Divide batter between loaf pans and bake at 350 degrees for 55 minutes. Remove from pans. Sprinkle with orange peel and powdered sugar while warm.

SERVING SIZE: 1 slice

CALORIES: 125   CHOL.: 1 mg.   FAT: 5 g.   SODIUM: 31 mg.

* = Dangerous to Some   ** = Consume with Caution   (see Pages 22 & 23)

# Confetti Muffins

**Makes 12 muffins**

**Prepare Ahead**
**\*\*Raspberries, nuts, lemon peel**

*A quick bread and easy to make. Remember; tip muffins to one side in pan, to prevent the bottom from getting steamy.*

NON-STICK COOKING SPRAY
1 cup FLOUR
2 tsp. BAKING POWDER
1 tsp. CINNAMON
2 EGG WHITES
1 cup fresh (or frozen unsweetened) RASPBERRIES\*\*
1/2 cup light MARGARINE
1/2 cup SKIM MILK
1/2 cup OAT BRAN
1/4 cup GRANULATED SUGAR
1/4 cup firmly packed BROWN SUGAR
1/4 tsp. SALT
1 tsp. LEMON PEEL\*\*, grated

## Nut Topping

In small bowl, combine 1/3 cup firmly packed brown sugar, 1/4 cup chopped nuts\*\*, 1/4 cup flour, 1 tablespoon light margarine and 1/2 teaspoon cinnamon. Mix with fork until crumbly. Set aside.

## Muffins

Spray 12 (2-1/2 inch) muffin cups with cooking spray. In medium bowl combine flour, oat bran, sugars, baking powder, cinnamon and salt. In large bowl mix egg whites, margarine and milk until blended. Stir in flour mixture just until moistened. Fold in raspberries and lemon peel. (If frozen raspberries are used, they must be thawed and well drained.) Spoon batter into prepared muffin cups. Sprinkle each with *Nut Topping*. Bake in 350 degree oven 20 to 25 minutes or until lightly browned and firm to touch. Cool in pan on wire rack 5 minutes. Remove from pan.

SERVING SIZE: 1 muffin

CALORIES: 180    CHOL.: 0    FAT: 6 g.    SODIUM: 220 mg.

\* = Dangerous to Some    \*\* = Consume with Caution    (see Pages 22 & 23)

# Applesauce Spice Muffins

**Quick and Easy**

**Makes 12 muffins**

*Moist, luscious muffins—remember that over-beating the batter causes "tunnels" and a tougher product.*

1/2 cup WHOLE WHEAT FLOUR
1/2 cup ALL-PURPOSE FLOUR
1-1/2 tsp. CINNAMON
1 cup UNSWEETENED APPLESAUCE
1 tsp. BAKING SODA
1/3 cup VEGETABLE OIL
1/4 tsp. GROUND CLOVES
3/4 cup firmly packed BROWN SUGAR
1 EGG or 1/4 cup EGG SUBSTITUTE
NON-STICK COOKING SPRAY

## Cream Cheese Frosting

In small bowl with mixer at low speed, beat 1-1/2 ounces (3 tablespoons) low-fat cream cheese, 1 teaspoon milk and 1 cup confectioner's sugar until blended. Beat on high speed 1 minute or until smooth.

## Muffins

Spray 12 (2-1/2 inch) muffin cups with cooking spray. In small bowl combine flours, cinnamon, baking soda and cloves. In medium bowl with mixer at low speed, beat applesauce, brown sugar, oil and egg until smooth. Beat in flour mixture. Increase speed to medium-high; beat 30 seconds. Spoon into prepared muffin cups; bake in 350 degree oven 18 minutes or until lightly browned and firm to touch. Cool in pan on wire rack 5 minutes. Remove from pan, cool completely. Spread with *Cream Cheese Frosting.*

SERVING SIZE: 1 Frosted Muffin

CALORIES: 210    CHOL.: 20 mg.  FAT: 8 g.  SODIUM: 95 mg.

* = Dangerous to Some   ** = Consume with Caution   (see Pages 22 & 23)

# Quick "Chocolate" Muffins

**Makes about 18 muffins**

. **Quick and Easy**
*Vanilla extract

*The oil in this recipe helps to make the muffins tender and free from tunnels and peaking.*

1-1/2 cups **ALL-PURPOSE FLOUR**
1/2 tsp. **SALT**
1 tsp. **BAKING SODA**
1 cup **WATER**
1 tsp. **VANILLA EXTRACT***
1/4 cup **CAROB POWDER**
1 cup **SUGAR**
1/4 cup plus 2 Tbsp. **VEGETABLE OIL**
1 Tbsp. **WHITE VINEGAR**

Heat oven to 375 degrees. In medium mixing bowl, combine flour, sugar, carob powder, baking soda and salt. Add water, oil, vinegar and vanilla. Beat with mixer, wire whisk or wooden spoon until batter is smooth and ingredients are well blended. Pour batter into paper-lined muffin pans (2-1/2 inch in diameter), filling each 2/3 full. Bake 16 to 18 minutes or until wooden toothpick inserted in center comes out clean. Remove to wire rack, cool completely. (Frost if desired.)

SERVING SIZE: 1 muffin

CALORIES: 129    CHOL.: 0    FAT: 5 g.    SODIUM: 121 mg.

* = Dangerous to Some    ** = Consume with Caution    (see Pages 22 & 23)

# Whole Grain Muffins

**Makes 12 muffins**

*These muffins aren't just tasty, they're nutritious, too. The oats and oat bran are also cholesterol-lowering agents.*

**1-1/2 cups SKIM MILK**
**1 Tbsp. plus 1 tsp. VEGETABLE OIL**
**1 cup QUICK-COOKING or REGULAR ROLLED OATS**
**ARTIFICIAL BROWN SUGAR equivalent to 1/4 cup sugar**
**3/4 cup uncooked OAT BRAN CEREAL**
**1 cup WHOLE WHEAT FLOUR**
**1 Tbsp. BAKING POWDER**
**1/4 cup EGG SUBSTITUTE, or 1 EGG**
**NON-STICK VEGETABLE SPRAY**

Heat oven to 400 degrees. Spray 12 (2-1/2-inch) muffin cups with non-stick vegetable spray, or line each with a paper baking cup. In a medium bowl, combine milk and oat bran cereal. Add egg substitute, brown sugar substitute and oil. Mix well. In a small bowl, combine remaining ingredients. Add to oat bran mixture. Mix until dry ingredients are moistened. Spoon into prepared muffin cups, filling until 2/3 full. Bake about 20 minutes or until light brown.

SERVING SIZE: 1 muffin

CALORIES: 103   CHOL.: 1 mg. FAT: 3.3 g. SODIUM: 132 mg.

* = Dangerous to Some   ** = Consume with Caution   (see Pages 22 & 23)

# French Coffee Cake

**Prepare Ahead**
***Vanilla extract**
****Yogurt, nuts**

**Makes 24 servings**

*Try this for a late evening snack, breakfast, or guests; inexpensive. The nuts can be omitted without hurting the flavor!*

1-1/4 cups SUGAR
1 cup DIET MARGARINE
1-1/2 tsp. VANILLA EXTRACT*
2 cups PLAIN NONFAT YOGURT**
1-1/2 tsp. BAKING POWDER
3 EGG WHITES
1 tsp. BAKING SODA
3 cups FLOUR
COOKING SPRAY

## Nut Filling

1/2 cup chopped WALNUTS** or PECANS**
1/4 cup firmly packed BROWN SUGAR
1/4 cup GRANULATED SUGAR
1-1/2 teaspoons CINNAMON

In small bowl combine filling ingredients. Mix with a fork until crumbly. Set aside.

## Coffee Cake

Spray 10-inch Bundt or 10 x 4-inch tube pan with cooking spray. In medium bowl with mixer at medium speed beat margarine and sugar until fluffy. Add yogurt, egg whites and vanilla; mix thoroughly. Combine flour, baking powder and baking soda. Gradually add to yogurt mixture, mixing well. Pour 1/3 of the batter into prepared pan. Sprinkle with half the *Nut Filling*. Repeat layers, ending with batter.

Bake in 350 degree oven 65 minutes or until toothpick inserted in center of cake comes out clean. Cool completely in pan on wire rack.

SERVING SIZE: 1/4 inch slice

CALORIES: 180    CHOL.: 0    FAT: 5 g.    SODIUM: 160 mg.

\* = Dangerous to Some    ** = Consume with Caution    (see Pages 22 & 23)

# French Toast

Quick and Easy
*Vanilla extract

*An old-time favorite with young and old that we often forget for breakfast variety.*

1 (8 oz.) carton EGG SUBSTITUTE, or 4 EGGS, beaten
1 tsp. GROUND CINNAMON
1 tsp. VANILLA EXTRACT*
1/3 cup SKIM MILK
10 slices LOW-SODIUM WHITE BREAD
2 Tbsp. MARGARINE
MAPLE FLAVORED SYRUP, optional

In shallow bowl, combine egg substitute, milk, cinnamon and vanilla.

In non-stick skillet, over medium heat, melt 2 teaspoons margarine. Dip bread slices in egg substitute mixture to coat; transfer to skillet. Brown about 3 minutes on each side, adding remaining margarine to skillet as needed. Serve with syrup, if desired.

SERVING SIZE: 2 slices (without syrup)

CALORIES: 189    CHOL.: 0    FAT: 6 g.        SODIUM: 121 mg.

* = Dangerous to Some    ** = Consume with Caution    (see Pages 22 & 23)

# Fruit Blintzes

Makes 16 blintzes

*An ethnic specialty to try for a change from the ordinary.*

**3/4 cup SKIM MILK**
**1 cup ALL-PURPOSE FLOUR**
**1/3 cup MARGARINE**
**1 (16 oz.) can sliced PEACHES packed in juice, well**
**drained and diced**
**1/2 cup chopped cooked PRUNES\***
**1 cup EGG SUBSTITUTE, or 4 EGGS**

Alternately add skim milk and flour to egg substitute, mixing until well combined.

Melt 1 teaspoon margarine; use to lightly grease a 6-inch skillet. Heat skillet; pour in a thin covering of prepared batter (about 2 tablespoons) just to cover bottom of pan. Tilt pan from side to side to distribute batter evenly. Cook on one side until batter blisters. Turn out onto a clean cloth or waxed paper. Repeat with remaining batter to make 16 blintzes, using melted margarine as needed.

Combine peaches and prunes. Place 1 tablespoonful of mixture on each blintz. Fold in sides to form a square. Melt 2 tablespoons margarine in a large skillet. Brown squares on both sides. Serve hot.

SERVING SIZE: 1 blintz

CALORIES: 91    CHOL.: 0    FAT: 4 g.    SODIUM: 59 mg.

\* = Dangerous to Some    \*\* = Consume with Caution    (see Pages 22 & 23)

# Gingerbread Raisin Pancakes

Makes 4 servings

*If you like ginger, you'll appreciate these pancakes. Like muffins, over-stirring causes a tougher product—the first pancakes prepared are the most tender.*

1-1/4 cup FLOUR
1/2 tsp. SALT
1/4 tsp. GROUND GINGER
1/3 cup RAISINS*
1 EGG
3 Tbsp. MARGARINE, melted
1/2 tsp. BAKING SODA
1/2 tsp. CINNAMON
1/4 cup MOLASSES
1 tsp. BAKING POWDER
1 cup SKIM MILK
NON-STICK COOKING SPRAY

In medium bowl combine flour, baking powder, baking soda, salt, cinnamon and ginger.

In small bowl mix egg, milk, molasses and margarine until blended. Add egg mixture to flour mixture, stirring just until moistened. Stir in raisins.

Spray griddle with cooking spray; heat. For each pancake, pour scant 1/4 cup batter onto hot griddle. Cook over medium heat, turning once, 4 minutes or until browned.

SERVING SIZE: 3 (4-inch) pancakes

CALORIES: 350   CHOL.: 55 mg.   FAT: 10 g.   SODIUM: 590 mg.

* = Dangerous to Some   ** = Consume with Caution   (see Pages 22 & 23)

# Jam Toast Triangles

### Quick and Easy
### Makes 5 servings

*A juicy, easy-to-make breakfast or supper dish enjoyed by both children and adults.*

**10 tsp. PRESERVES or JAM, any flavor except raspberry, orange or fig**
**1/4 cup EGG SUBSTITUTE, or 1 EGG**
**2 Tbsp. MARGARINE**
**1/4 cup SKIM MILK**
**5 slices BREAD**
**1/4 tsp. GROUND CINNAMON**
**1 Tbsp. SUGAR**

Spread 2 teaspoons preserves onto each slice of bread. Cut each slice diagonally in half. Place one half over the other to form a sandwich; press to seal.

In medium bowl, combine egg substitute and skim milk. Dip each sandwich in egg mixture to coat. In medium skillet, over medium-high heat, melt margarine. Add sandwiches; cook until toasted on both sides.

Combine sugar and cinnamon; sprinkle over top; serve warm.

SERVING SIZE: 2 triangles

CALORIES: 166     CHOL.: 1 mg.     FAT: 5 g.     SODIUM: 285 mg.

* = Dangerous to Some     ** = Consume with Caution     (see Pages 22 & 23)

# Vegetable Omelet

*A quick-to-prepare omelet with colorful vegetables and no cholesterol. Use egg substitute, 1/2 cup, if preferred.*

**1/4 cup EGG SUBSTITUTE**
**2 Tbsp. finely diced RED or GREEN PEPPER**
**3 Tbsp. finely diced BROCCOLI**
**1 tsp. finely diced ONION** or chives**
**1 tsp. OLIVE OIL**
**SALT and PEPPER to taste**

Combine olive oil, broccoli, pepper and onion in frying pan. Cook over medium heat for about 2 minutes, stirring constantly. Pour egg substitute over vegetables and cook until thickened but still moist. Serve immediately.

SERVING SIZE: 1 omelet

CALORIES: 84    CHOL.: 0    FAT: 4.6 g.    SODIUM: 115 mg.

* = Dangerous to Some    ** = Consume with Caution    (see Pages 22 & 23)

# Omelet Primavera

**Makes 2 servings**

*Omelets seem to make any meal special. They are suitable for a summer luncheon or evening meal as well as breakfast.*

**1/2 cup sliced YELLOW SQUASH**
**1/2 cup sliced ZUCCHINI**
**1/4 cup RED PEPPER STRIPS**
**1/4 cup GREEN PEPPER STRIPS**
**2 tsp. MARGARINE**
**1 cup sliced MUSHROOMS***
**1 container (7.5 oz.) EGG SUBSTITUTE**

Melt 1 teaspoon margarine in an 8-inch non-stick omelet pan, over medium heat. Add vegetables; cook and stir until tender-crisp. Remove from pan; set aside. In same pan, melt remaining margarine; pour in egg substitute. Cook, lifting edges to allow uncooked portion to flow underneath. When almost set, spoon vegetables over half of omelet. With spatula, fold other half over filling; slide onto serving dish. Serve immediately.

SERVING SIZE: 1/2 omelet

CALORIES: 112    CHOL.: 0    FAT: 4 g.    SODIUM: 120 mg.

---

* = Dangerous to Some    ** = Consume with Caution    (see Pages 22 & 23)

# Breakfast Burrito

**Quick and Easy**
**Makes 1 serving**

*A south-of-the-border change from the usual breakfast*

**1/2 cup EGG SUBSTITUTE, or 2 EGGS**
**1 CORN TORTILLA**
**VEGETABLE COOKING SPRAY**
**2 Tbsp. CHUNKY SALSA (mild, medium or hot)**

Spray non-stick skillet with vegetable spray; pour egg substitute in skillet and cook to desired doneness. Microwave corn tortilla for 30 seconds. Fill tortilla with cooked egg substitute. Top with salsa.

MICROWAVE: Pour egg substitute into small microwave-safe bowl. Cook on MEDIUM (60-70% power) for 1 minute or until desired doneness. Microwave corn tortilla for 30 seconds. Fill tortilla with cooked egg substitute. Top with salsa.

SERVING SIZE: 1 burrito

CALORIES: 92     CHOL.: 0     FAT: 1 g.     SODIUM: 340 mg.

* = Dangerous to Some    ** = Consume with Caution    (see Pages 22 & 23)

# Egg Salad on Bagels

**Quick and Easy**
**\*Mayonnaise (check label)**
**\*\*Yogurt**

**Makes 4 servings**

*Skip the top half of the bagel to lower the calories.*

1 tsp. DIJON MUSTARD
1 Tbsp. "light" MAYONNAISE\* (check label)
4 hard-cooked EGG WHITES, chopped
4 whole BAGELS, sliced horizontally
1/2 cup PLAIN NONFAT YOGURT\*\*
1/4 cup chopped CELERY
1/4 tsp. DILL WEED
1 hard-cooked EGG YOLK, chopped

In medium bowl, combine all ingredients except eggs and bagels. Add egg whites and yolk, fold in gently.

Spread 1/3 cup of mixture on each of 4 bagel halves. Top with remaining bagel halves.

SERVING SIZE: 1 salad bagel

CALORIES: 229   CHOL.: 70 mg.   FAT: 4 g.   SODIUM: 4 mg.

\* = Dangerous to Some   \*\* = Consume with Caution   (see Pages 22 & 23)

# Toasted Egg Salad Sandwiches

Makes 6 servings

Quick and Easy
**Scallions

*An old favorite minus the cholesterol.*

2 cartons (8 oz.) EGG SUBSTITUTE
1/4 cup CREAMY MAYONNAISE *(see Salads, Salad Dressings)*
12 slices LOW-SODIUM WHITE BREAD
1/4 cup chopped CELERY
1/4 cup chopped RED PEPPER
2 Tbsp. chopped SCALLIONS**
6 LETTUCE LEAVES

In large non-stick skillet, pour egg substitute; cover tightly; cook over very low heat 10 minutes or just until set. Remove from heat; let stand, covered, for 10 minutes. Remove from skillet; cool completely; coarsely chop.

In bowl, combine hard cooked egg substitute, mayonnaise, celery, red pepper and scallions. Cover; chill until serving time. Divide and spread on 6 toasted bread slices; top with lettuce and remaining bread. Serve immediately.

SERVING SIZE: 1 sandwich

CALORIES: 238    CHOL. 0        FAT: 8 g.   SODIUM: 127 mg.

---

* = Dangerous to Some    ** = Consume with Caution    (see Pages 22 & 23)

# Desserts, Sweets

# Baked Apple Crumble

**Easy**

**Makes 8 servings**  **Orange juice, yogurt (optional)

*Another old-fashioned favorite you may have known as Apple Betty. Instead of baking in an oiled casserole, a pie shell can be substituted if you prefer pastry.*

## Apple layer

**6 cups sliced, peeled APPLES (about 2 lbs. or 6 medium apples)**
**2 Tbsp. ORANGE JUICE** or other fruit juice**
**3 Tbsp. VEGETABLE OIL**
**3/4 cup firmly packed LIGHT SUGAR**
**1/2 cup ALL-PURPOSE FLOUR**
**1/2 tsp. CINNAMON**

## Topping

(optional)

**1/2 cup VANILLA LOW-FAT YOGURT**, divided**

Heat oven to 375 degrees. Oil 2-quart casserole or baking dish. Arrange apples evenly in dish. Drizzle with orange juice.

Combine sugar, flour and cinnamon. Mix in oil until crumbly. Spoon over apples.

Bake at 375 degrees for 35 minutes or until apples are tender. Cool slightly; serve warm.

For optional topping, spoon one tablespoon vanilla yogurt over each serving.

SERVING SIZE: 2/3 cup

CALORIES: 200    CHOL.: 0   FAT: 6 g.   SODIUM: 10 mg.

* = Dangerous to Some   ** = Consume with Caution   (see Pages 22 & 23)

# Banana Cream Pie

**Prepare Ahead**
***Vanilla extract**

Makes 10 servings

****Bananas**

*Your family or guest may go ape over this pie and only you know that the sugar-free pudding mix, skim milk and low-calorie topping mix help with the calorie count.*

## Crust

7 large GRAHAM CRACKERS, crumbled
3 Tbsp. MARGARINE, melted
2 packets SWEETENER

Combine graham cracker crumbs, margarine and sweetener in a small bowl. Using the back of a spoon, press crumb mixture into a 9-inch pie plate. Chill 3 hours or more.

## Filling

1 4-serving size INSTANT SUGAR-FREE VANILLA
    PUDDING MIX
1 envelope REDUCED-CALORIE WHIPPED TOPPING MIX
2 cups SKIM MILK
1/2 tsp. VANILLA EXTRACT*
3 medium BANANAS** (not overly ripe)

Prepare pudding according to package directions. Chill until slightly thickened. In a separate bowl, prepare whipped topping mix according to package directions. Add vanilla. Fold topping into pudding. Slice bananas and arrange in pie crust. Top with pudding mixture. Chill several hours before serving.

SERVING SIZE: 1/10 of pie.

CALORIES: 165   CHOL.: 0   FAT: 6 g.   SODIUM: 276 mg.

* = Dangerous to Some   ** = Consume with Caution   (see Pages 22 & 23)

# Banana Snacking Cake

**Makes 24 servings**

**Prepare Ahead**
**\*\*Bananas, walnuts, yogurt**

*Note that this moist cake is cholesterol-free. Avoid bananas that are over-ripe; they contain more of the blood pressure agent, tyramine.*

2-1/4 cups ALL-PURPOSE FLOUR
1-1/4 cup mashed BANANAS\*\* (about 2 large)
1/3 cup MARGARINE, softened
1-1/4 cups SUGAR
3/4 cup EGG SUBSTITUTE, or 3 EGGS
2 tsp. BAKING POWDER
1 tsp. BAKING SODA
2/3 cup PLAIN NONFAT YOGURT\*\*
1/2 cup WALNUTS\*\*, chopped (optional)
CONFECTIONER'S SUGAR (optional)

In small bowl, combine flour, baking powder and baking soda; set aside.

In large bowl, with electric mixer at medium speed, beat margarine and white sugar until well combined. At low speed, blend in egg substitute and bananas. Add flour mixture alternately with yogurt, mixing until smooth. Stir in walnuts, if desired.

Spoon batter into greased and floured 13 x 9 x 2-inch baking pan. Bake at 350 degrees for 45 minutes, or until toothpick inserted in center comes out clean. Cool in pan on wire rack. Dust with confectioner's sugar, if desired, before serving.

SERVING SIZE: 2 x 2 inch squares

CALORIES: 129    CHOL.: 0    FAT: 3 g.    SODIUM: 98 mg.

* = Dangerous to Some    ** = Consume with Caution    (see Pages 22 & 23)

# Brown Edge Wafers

Makes 4 dozen

Prepare Ahead
*Vanilla extract
**Lemon rind

*These are similar to the vanilla wafers so popular on super-market shelves; they also taste like un-iced Christmas cookies.*

1/2 cup MARGARINE
1/2 cup SUGAR
1/4 tsp. grated LEMON RIND**
3 Tbsp. EGG SUBSTITUTE, or 1 EGG
1 tsp. VANILLA EXTRACT*
1 cup ALL-PURPOSE FLOUR

In small bowl of electric mixer, cream margarine and sugar until light and fluffy. Beat in egg substitute, vanilla and lemon rind until smooth. Gradually add flour, beating until well blended.

Drop dough by teaspoonsful onto greased baking sheets; flatten slightly. Bake at 375 degrees for 7 minutes or until done. Carefully remove from baking sheets and cool on wire racks.

SERVING SIZE: 2 wafers

CALORIES: 35    CHOL.: 0    FAT: 2 g.    SODIUM: 18 mg.

* = Dangerous to Some    ** = Consume with Caution    (see Pages 22 & 23)

# Cannoli Cream

Quick and Easy
Prepare Ahead
*Raisins

Makes 8 servings          **Rum extract, orange marmalade

*This creamy, yet crunchy, dessert supplies good nutrition in that important mineral, calcium. Be sure the raisins are fresh—less likely to instigate a headache!*

1 lb. part-SKIM RICOTTA or COTTAGE CHEESE
1/4 cup SKIM MILK
1/2 tsp. RUM EXTRACT**
1/3 cup soft GOLDEN RAISINS*
1/4 cup slivered MACADAMIA NUTS
1/4 cup ORANGE MARMALADE**

In a blender or food processor, whir ricotta cheese, milk, marmalade and rum flavoring until smooth. Stir in raisins. Refrigerate 1 hour or longer. Stir in macadamia nuts before serving. Divide mixture among 8 stemmed glasses.

SERVING SIZE: 3/4 cup

CALORIES: 159   CHOL.: 3 mg.   FAT: 7 g.   SODIUM: 83 mg.

* = Dangerous to Some   ** = Consume with Caution   (see Pages 22 & 23)

# Caramel Custard with Egg Substitute

Makes 6 servings

Prepare Ahead
*Vanilla extract

*This popular custard, served around the world, can be served in the custard cups without inverting over individual plates.*

6 Tbsp. SUGAR
3/4 cup EGG SUBSTITUTE, or 3 EGGS, beaten
2-2/3 cups SKIM MILK, scalded
1/3 cup SUGAR
3/4 tsp. VANILLA EXTRACT*

Preheat oven to 350 degrees. Melt 6 tablespoons sugar in a small skillet over low to medium heat until golden brown; pour at once into 6 (6 oz.) heatproof custard cups. Tilt dishes to coat evenly; set aside.

Scald milk (heat milk in saucepan over low heat until bubbles form around the edges). Combine egg substitute and 1/3 cup sugar; stir in scalded milk and vanilla; slowly pour into custard cups. Set cups in a shallow baking pan filled 1-inch deep with hot water. Bake at 350 degrees for 25 to 30 minutes or until a knife inserted in center comes out clean; cool to room temperature. Chill 2 hours or until firm.

To serve, loosen edges with a knife and invert over individual plates.

SERVING SIZE: 1/2 cup

CALORIES: 139    CHOL.: 2 mg.    FAT: 1 g.    SODIUM: 107 mg.

* = Dangerous to Some    ** = Consume with Caution    (see Pages 22 & 23)

# Carrot Cake

*A lower-calorie, moist, easy-to-prepare favorite.*

1 cup grated CARROTS
1/2 cup chopped MACADAMIA NUTS
2/3 cup SWEETENER
1 tsp. BAKING SODA
1/2 tsp. CINNAMON
1/2 cup VEGETABLE OIL
1/2 cup RAISINS* (fresh, not aged)
2 EGGS
1 cup FLOUR
1/2 tsp. SALT

Grease 8 x 8-inch glass pan. Combine sweetener, vegetable oil and eggs in a bowl and beat until blended. Add flour, baking soda, cinnamon, salt, grated carrots, chopped nuts and raisins. Stir well. Pour mixture in pan. Bake at 350 degrees for 35 to 40 minutes. Allow to cool completely before frosting.

**Frosting**
6 oz. CREAM CHEESE
1/2 tsp. COCONUT EXTRACT*
3 packets of SWEETENER
1/2 tsp. VANILLA EXTRACT*

Combine ingredients in a bowl and blend well.

SERVING SIZE: 2 x 2 inch square

CALORIES: 138   CHOL.: 34 mg.  FAT: 10 g. SODIUM: 157 mg.

* = Dangerous to Some   ** = Consume with Caution   (see Pages 22 & 23)

# Cashew Raisin Nuggets

**Prepare Ahead**
***Raisins, vanilla extract**
****Cashews**

**Makes 3 dozen cookies**

*These cookies are tasty and never seem to dry out, even when frozen for two weeks!*

1-1/2 cups WHOLE WHEAT FLOUR
1/2 cup MARGARINE
3 Tbsp. EGG SUBSTITUTE, or 1 EGG
1/2 cup chopped, dry roasted, unsalted CASHEWS**
1/4 tsp. GROUND CINNAMON
1/2 cup SUGAR
1 tsp. VANILLA EXTRACT*
1/4 cup SKIM MILK
1/2 cup DARK SEEDLESS RAISINS*

Combine flour and cinnamon; set aside. Cream together margarine and sugar on medium speed of electric mixer. Beat in egg substitute and vanilla until light and creamy. Blend flour mixture and skim milk alternately into creamed mixture until smooth. Stir in cashews and raisins.

Drop mixture by rounded teaspoonful onto ungreased baking sheets. Bake at 375 degrees for 10 minutes or until done. Remove cookies from sheets and cool on wire racks.

SERVING SIZE: 1 cookie

CALORIES: 68     CHOL.: 0          FAT: 3 g.   SODIUM: 25 mg.

* = Dangerous to Some   ** = Consume with Caution   (see Pages 22 & 23)

# "Chocolate" Pudding Parfaits

**Makes 8 servings**

Prepare Ahead
*Vanilla extract
**Orange slices, orange peel

*A very pretty dessert that can be made ahead of time to top off any luncheon or dinner.*

2/3 cup SUGAR
1/2 cup cold SKIM MILK
1/4 tsp. grated ORANGE PEEL**
2 cups SKIM MILK
1 envelope (1.4 oz.) WHIPPED TOPPING MIX
1/4 cup CAROB POWDER
1 tsp. VANILLA EXTRACT*
1/4 tsp. VANILLA EXTRACT*
1 Tbsp. MARGARINE
3 Tbsp. CORNSTARCH
dash SALT
ORANGE SLICES**, optional

In medium saucepan combine sugar, carob powder, cornstarch and salt; gradually stir in 2 cups skim milk. Cook over medium heat, stirring constantly, until mixture boils; boil and stir 1 minute. Remove from heat; blend in margarine and 1 teaspoon vanilla. Pour into medium bowl. Press plastic wrap onto surface of pudding; chill.

In small bowl combine topping mix, 1/2 cup cold skim milk and 1/4 teaspoon vanilla; prepare according to package directions. Fold 1/2 cup whipped topping into pudding. Blend orange peel into remaining whipped topping.

Alternately spoon "chocolate" pudding and orange flavored whipped topping into parfait glasses. Chill. Garnish with orange slices, if desired.

SERVING SIZE: 2/3 cup

CALORIES: 176    CHOL.: 2 mg.    FAT: 4 g.    SODIUM: 93 mg.

* = Dangerous to Some    ** = Consume with Caution    (see Pages 22 & 23)

# Elegant "Chocolate" Angel Torte

Makes 16 servings

Prepare Ahead
*Vanilla extract

*Make this "heavenly" dessert ahead of time. Some markets carry carob powder, but almost all health stores have it on their shelves.*

1/3 cup CAROB POWDER
1 tsp. VANILLA EXTRACT*
2 pkgs. (4 oz.) (2 envelopes) WHIPPED TOPPING MIX
1 cup cold SKIM MILK
STRAWBERRIES to make 1 cup STRAWBERRY PURÉE
1 pkg. (14.5 oz.) ANGEL FOOD CAKE mix, or one
    purchased cake
STRAWBERRIES

Combine carob powder and contents of cake flour packet. Proceed with mixing cake as directed on package. Bake and cool as directed. Slice cooled cake crosswise (horizontally) into four 1-inch slices.

In large mixer bowl combine topping mix, cold milk and vanilla; prepare according to package directions. Blend in strawberry puree. Place bottom cake slice on serving plate; spread with 1/4 of topping. Stack next cake layer; spread with topping. Continue layering cake and topping. Garnish with strawberries. Refrigerate.

To serve, use sharp serrated knife and cut vertically with a gentle sawing motion.

SERVING SIZE: 1/16 of cake

CALORIES: 154     CHOL.: 0     FAT: 2 g.     SODIUM: 73 mg.

* = Dangerous to Some     ** = Consume with Caution     (see Pages 22 & 23)

# Fudgy Brownies

Quick and Easy
Prepare Ahead
*Vanilla extract
**Walnuts

Makes 16 servings

*In this recipe the margarine may be melted in a heavy sauce-pan and when just warm, add all the other ingredients— quick and easy, and a very special treat.*

1/4 cup MARGARINE
1/2 cup firmly packed LIGHT BROWN SUGAR
1/4 cup WALNUTS**, chopped
1 tsp. VANILLA EXTRACT*
1/2 cup SUGAR
1/2 cup ALL-PURPOSE FLOUR
2 Tbsp. CAROB POWDER
3 Tbsp. EGG SUBSTITUTE, or 1 EGG

Melt margarine. In a large bowl or heavy saucepan combine margarine, sugars, flour, carob powder and egg substitute until well blended. Stir in vanilla extract and walnuts. Spread batter evenly in a well-greased 8 x 8 x 2-inch baking pan.

Bake at 350 degrees for 30 minutes or until tests baked. Cool in pan on wire rack. Cut into 2-inch squares while warm.

SERVING SIZE: 2 x 2 inch square

CALORIES: 105     CHOL.: 0     FAT: 4 g.     SODIUM: 31 mg.

* = Dangerous to Some    ** = Consume with Caution    (see Pages 22 & 23)

# Glazed Apple Tart

Makes 10 servings

Prepare Ahead
**Orange marmalade

*The glaze on the apple tart gives a professional appearance.*

6 Tbsp. SUGAR
1/4 tsp. GROUND CINNAMON
1 Tbsp. MARGARINE
1/2 cup ORANGE MARMALADE**
1 Tbsp. CORNSTARCH
6 cups (about 3 large) thickly sliced pared baking APPLES
*Single Crust Flaky Pastry* (see *Desserts, Sweets*)

Roll out pastry to a 12 inch circle. Fit into a 9-inch springform pan or pie plate, making edges 3/4-inch high.

Mix sugar, cornstarch, cinnamon and apple slices. Overlap apple slices in a circular pattern in prepared pastry. Dot with margarine. Cover with foil. Bake at 400 degrees for 45 minutes.

Heat marmalade over low heat just until thin. Uncover tart and drizzle over apples. Continue baking tart, uncovered, 15 minutes longer or until apples are tender. Cool.

SERVING SIZE: 1/10 of tart

CALORIES: 230    CHOL.: 0    FAT: 7 g.    SODIUM: 62 mg.

* = Dangerous to Some    ** = Consume with Caution    (see Pages 22 & 23)

# Honey Walnut Cake

## (Lekach)

**Makes 9 servings**

*These bars freeze well and will satisfy anyone's sweet tooth.*

1/2 cup firmly packed LIGHT BROWN SUGAR
1/4 cup EGG SUBSTITUTE, or 1 EGG
1 tsp. INSTANT COFFEE POWDER*
1/4 tsp. GROUND ALLSPICE
1/4 cup SKIM MILK
1/2 cup MARGARINE
1/2 cup HONEY
1 cup ALL-PURPOSE FLOUR
1/4 tsp. BAKING SODA
1/4 tsp. GROUND CINNAMON
1/4 tsp. GROUND CLOVES
1/4 cup WALNUTS**, chopped

Cream together margarine, brown sugar and honey. Add egg substitute and continue beating until mixture is fluffy. Mix in flour, instant coffee, baking soda, cinnamon, cloves, allspice, skim milk and walnuts until well blended.

Spread batter in a greased 8-inch square baking pan. Bake at 375 degrees for 30 minutes or until done. Cool in pan on wire rack. Cut into 9 pieces.

SERVING SIZE: 2-1/2 inch square

CALORIES: 270   CHOL.: 0   FAT: 12 g.   SODIUM: 125 mg.

* = Dangerous to Some   ** = Consume with Caution   (see Pages 22 & 23)

# Lemon Love Notes

Prepare Ahead—Gourmet
*Vanilla extract
Makes approx. 20 bars bars  *Lemon juice, lemon rind

*A wonderfully tart and delicious treat. An old-fashioned favorite handed down through generations.*

Crust:
   1/2 cup MARGARINE
   1/4 cup POWDERED SUGAR
   1 cup FLOUR

Mix well with pastry blender or fork. Put into well-greased 8-inch square pan, lined with greased brown paper. Bake 15 minutes at 350 degrees.

Filling:
   2 Tbsp. LEMON JUICE**
   1/2 cup EGG SUBSTITUTE, or 2 EGGS, beaten well
   1/2 tsp. BAKING POWDER
   1/2 cup SUGAR
   2 Tbsp. FLOUR
   Grated fresh rind of 1 LEMON**

Mix above ingredients well and beat. Place on just baked crust; return to 350 degree oven and bake 25 minutes. Cool and frost with:

Thin Icing:
   3/4 cup POWDERED SUGAR
   1/2 tsp. VANILLA EXTRACT*
   1 Tbsp. MARGARINE
   2 tsp. MILK

Combine and spread over bars.

SERVING SIZE: 1 bar (1-1/2 by 2 inches ea.)

CALORIES: 73   CHOL.: 0   FAT: 3 g.   SODIUM: 33 mg.

* = Dangerous to Some   ** = Consume with Caution   (see Pages 22 & 23)

# Mock Rice Pudding

**Makes 6 servings**

Prepare Ahead
**Mandarin oranges, peach yogurt

*This recipe, with three fruit ingredients, can nutritionally "sweeten" your everyday menu.*

1 can (10-11 oz.) MANDARIN ORANGES**, drained
1 can (10-12 oz.) crushed PINEAPPLE, drained
1 APPLE, cored, diced
2 cups cooked WHITE RICE
1 carton (8 oz.) LOW-FAT PEACH YOGURT**

Combine all ingredients in bowl, mix. Refrigerate until serving time.

SERVING SIZE: 3/4 cup

CALORIES: 184    CHOL.: 2 mg.    FAT: 1 g.    SODIUM: 60 mg.

# Saucepan Butterscotch Brownies

Prepare Ahead
*Vanilla extract
**Makes 24 bars (1-1/2 x 3 inches)**                    **Nuts

*A rich, satisfying "brownie" that truly fulfills that sweet-tooth longing. Admittedly an indulgence for special occasions.*

1 stick (or 1/2 cup) MARGARINE
1-1/2 cups BROWN SUGAR, packed
1-1/2 cups sifted FLOUR
2 EGGS (or 1/2 cup EGG SUBSTITUTE)
1 tsp. VANILLA EXTRACT*
2 tsp. BAKING SODA
1 cup chopped NUTS**

Grease 9 x 13-inch pan. Melt margarine in a saucepan. Remove from heat. Add sugar and blend. Add eggs, beating well. Stir in vanilla, flour and baking powder. Pour into prepared pan. Bake in a 350 degree oven about 30 minutes. Do not overbake. Cool in pan and then cut into bars.

SERVING SIZE: 1 bar

CALORIES: 115    CHOL.: 0         FAT: 5 g.    SODIUM: 98 mg.

* = Dangerous to Some    ** = Consume with Caution    (see Pages 22 & 23)

# Savannah Peach Melba

**Prepare Ahead**
***Vanilla extract**
****Raspberries**

**Makes 4 servings**

*This dessert can be made ahead of time. Guests will ask for the recipe.*

**1 pkg. (3-3/8 oz.) INSTANT VANILLA PUDDING & PIE FILLING, or 1 pkg. (1.7 oz.) SUGAR-FREE INSTANT VANILLA PUDDING & PIE FILLING***
**2 Tbsp. prepared WHIPPED TOPPING (for garnish)**
**1 cup fresh or frozen RASPBERRIES**, pureed**
**2 cups cold SKIM MILK**
**1 can (8 oz.) PEACHES, drained and chopped**
**RASPBERRIES** and MINT LEAVES, for garnish**

In medium bowl, prepare pudding according to package directions, using skim milk. Stir in peaches. In 4 glasses (8 oz.) layer pudding mixture and raspberry puree. Chill at least 1 hour. To serve, garnish with whipped topping, raspberries and mint, if desired.

SERVING SIZE: 5 oz.

CALORIES: 267    CHOL.: 10 mg.  FAT: 3 g.  SODIUM: 246 mg.

# Single Crust Flaky Pastry

**Prepare Ahead**
**Makes one 9-inch crust**

*No salt is provided in this recipe (for those on low sodium), so add 1 / 8 teaspoon salt to the flour, if desired.*

**1/3 cup MARGARINE**
**3-4 Tbsp. ICE WATER**
**1-1/4 cups ALL-PURPOSE FLOUR**

Cut margarine into flour with pastry cutter or 2 forks until mixture resembles coarse meal. Add 3 to 4 tablespoons ice water, a tablespoon at a time, tossing until moistened. Shape into a ball. Pastry can be chilled until ready to use. Place dough between 2 pieces waxed paper. Roll to fit a 9-inch pie pan.

Nutritional value included in recipes using this pie crust.

* = Dangerous to Some   ** = Consume with Caution   (see Pages 22 & 23)

# Smorgasbord Cheesecake

**Prepare Ahead**
**Gourmet**
***Vanilla extract**
****Sour cream**

**Makes 8 servings (1 loaf pan)**

*This truly delicious cheesecake is not exactly inexpensive, but is well worth the cost.*

1/2 lb. CREAM CHEESE
1/3 cup SUGAR
1/2 tsp. VANILLA EXTRACT*
1/4 cup EGG SUBSTITUTE, or 2 EGGS
Few grains SALT

Beat together well the above ingredients, pour into a loaf pan or an 8-inch pie pan. Bake 35 minutes at 275 degrees.

Top with a mixture of:

1/2 pint SOUR CREAM**
2-1/2 Tbsp. SUGAR
1/2 tsp. VANILLA EXTRACT*
Few grains SALT

Bake 7 minutes at 275 degrees. Refrigerate.

SERVING SIZE: 1/8 cake

CALORIES: 257   CHOL.: 31 mg.  FAT: 16 g. SODIUM: 189 mg.

* = Dangerous to Some   ** = Consume with Caution   (see Pages 22 & 23)

# FOOTNOTES

## INTRODUCTION

1. Plenge, Kathern, M.D.: *An Ounce of Prevention.* Barrows Neurological Institute, St. Joseph's Hospital and Medical Center, Phoenix, Arizona. Volume VI, Issue 3, 1991.

2. New York, New York: *Wall Street Journal.* "Drug of Bristol-Myers to Treat Ovarian Cancer, Taxol, Approved." December 30, 1992.

3. "New Migraine Research," Phoenix, Arizona: *The Arizona Republic,* December 26, 1994.

## CHAPTER 1

1. McCarthy, Pam, R.D.: *Fleishmann's Cholesterol Management Program,* University of Minnesota School of Public Health, December 1, 1989.

2. Taber. Clarence Wilbur: *Taber's Cyclopedic Medical Dictionary* Philadelphia: F.A. Davis Company, 1985.

3. Hanington, E: *Preliminary Report on Tyramine Headaches.* Br. Med.J.2:550, 1967.

4. Brainard, John G: *Control of Migraine.* New York: W.W. Norton and Company, 1979.

5. Grasso, Patricia Holter and Stump, Jan Schaller: *The Headache Cookbook:* "A Tool For Migraine Self-Help." Bowie, Maryland: Robert J. Brady Company, 1984.

6. Solomon, Neil: Phoenix, Arizona: *Phoenix Newspapers, Inc.* March 15, August 25, September 1, 1990.

7. Blake, Joan Salge: "Can Migraines be Managed Through Diet? Food That May be to Blame." *Environmental Nutrition,* 11:1, 1988.

8. Stern, Loraine: "Sudden Pain - What Causes It, How to Relieve It; How to Prevent It; When to See a Doctor." Deamandis Communications, Inc. *Woman's Day Medical Facts Guide,* 1989.

9. Diamond, Seymour: "Headaches Can Be a Pain, But Can Be Prevented or Treated." *Diabetes in the News,* 9:3, 1990.

10. Wedman, Betty: *Diet and Meal Plans to Control Migraine Headaches.* Fort Atkinson, Wisconsin: NosCo, 1985.

11. Phoenix, Arizona: *Phoenix Newspapers, Inc.* "High Tension Show Turns Headaches into Artwork." August 6, 1990.

12. Webster, Guy: "Pain Pills May Add to Headache." Phoenix, Arizona: *Phoenix Newspapers, Inc.,* October 2, 1989.

## CHAPTER 2

1. Foundation for Research in Head Pain and Related Disorders, Dept. P, P.O. Box 5137, San Clemente, California, 92672.

2. Krause, Marie V. and Mahan, L. Kathleen: *Food Nutrition and Diet Therapy.* Philadelphia: W. B. Saunders Company,1984.

3. Powers, Dorothy E. and Moore, Ann O: *Food Medications Interactions.* Phoenix, Arizona: Food Medication Interactions, 1988.

4. Goodhart, Robert S. and Shils, Maurice E: *Modern Nutrition in Health and Disease.* New York, New York: Lea and Febiger, 1980.

5. Blake, Joan Salge: "Can Migraine Be Managed Through Diet? Foods That May Be to Blame." *Environmental Nutrition,* 11:1,1988.

6. Koehler, S. M. and Glaros, A: "The Effect of Aspartame on Migraine Headaches." *Headache,* 28:10, 1988.

## CHAPTER 3

1. Brainard, John B. *Control of Migraine,* New York, New York, W. W. Norton and Co., 1979.

2. Grasso, Patricia Holter and Stump, Jan Schaller: *The Headache Cookbook, A Tool for Migraine Self-Help.* Bowie, Maryland: Robert J. Brady Company, 1984.

3. Pappas, Nancy: "Dangerous liaisons: When Food and Drugs Don't Mix." Boulder, Colorado: *In Health,* July/August 1990

4. Griffith, H. Winter: *Complete Guide to Prescription and Non-Prescription Drugs.* Tucson, Arizona: HP Books, Inc., 1986.

5. Pennington, Jean A.T. and Church, Helen Nicholas: *Food Values of Portions Commonly Used.* New York, New York: Harper and Rowe, Publishers, 1985.

6. Powers, Dorothy E. and Moore, Ann O: *Food and Medication Interactions.* Phoenix, Arizona: Food Medication Interactions, 1988.

7. Webster, Guy: "Pain Pills May Add to Headaches." Phoenix, Arizona: *The Arizona Republic,* October 1, 1990.

8. "Healthwatch: Aspirin Regimen May Offer Migraine Relief." Washington, D.C: *A.A.R.P. Bulletin,* Vol. 31, No. 6.

9. Brackenridge, Betty Page, R.D. "How to Create a Super Supermarket Shopping Plan." South Bend, Indiana: *Diabetes in the News,* Vol.9, No.3, 1990.

10. "The Sodium Content of Your Food." *Home and Garden Bulletin* Number 233. Washington, D.C: U.S. Government Printing Office, 1982.

11. Alishire, Peter: "Fish Oil or Snake Oil?" Phoenix, Arizona: *The Arizona Republic,* July 22, 1990.

## CHAPTER 4, RECIPES AND TABLES

1. *New Light-Style Cooking.* Westbury; New York: Pam®, 1988.
2. *Diet for a Healthy Heart.* East Hanover, N. J: Nabisco Brands, Inc., 1988.
3. Pennington, A. T. and Church, Helen Nicholas: *Food Values of Portions Commonly Used.* New York: Harper and Row, Publishers, 1985.
4. *Nutrition in the Nineties - a Glance Back and a Glimpse Ahead. On Your Mark.* Washington, D.C: The Sugar Association, Inc., March 1990.
5. National Research Council. *Diet and Health Implications for Reducing Chronic Disease Risk.* Page 16. National Academy Press, Washington, D.C., 1989.
6. Allen, Ann Moore: Powers and Moore's *Food-Medication Interactions,* Tempe, Arizona: Ann Moore Allen, Publisher, 1991.
7. Arizona Dietetic Association, Inc.: *Arizona Diet Manual.* Phoenix, Arizona: Arizona Department of Health Services, Office of Nutrition Services, and Tucson, Arizona: University of Arizona, College of Medicine, Department of Family and Community Medicine, Health Services Section, 1992.
8. McCarthy, Pam, R.D: *Fleishmann's Cholesterol Management Program,* University of Minnesota School of Public Health, 1989.
9. *Eat Healthy America.* Coventry, CT: Best Foods, CPC International, Inc. 1990.

# INDEX